Menopause

Manage Its
Symptoms
with
the Blood
Type Diet®

Also by Dr. Peter J. D'Adamo with Catherine Whitney

Eat Right 4 Your Type: The Individualized Diet Solution to Staying Healthy, Living Longer, and Achieving Your Ideal Weight

Cook Right 4 Your Type: The Practical Kitchen Companion to Eat Right 4 Your Type

Live Right 4 Your Type: The Individualized Prescription for Maximizing Health, Metabolism, and Vitality in Every Stage of Your Life

Eat Right 4 Your Type Complete Blood Type Encyclopedia

Eat Right 4 Your Baby: The Individualized Guide to Fertility and Maximum Health During Pregnancy, Nursing, and Your Baby's First Year

Blood Type O: Food, Beverage and Supplement Lists

Blood Type A: Food, Beverage and Supplement Lists

Blood Type B: Food, Beverage and Supplement Lists

Blood Type AB: Food, Beverage and Supplement Lists

Dr. Peter J. D'Adamo Eat Right 4 (for) Your Type Health Library

Aging: Fight It with the Blood Type Diet®

Allergies: Fight Them with the Blood Type Diet®

Arthritis: Fight It with the Blood Type Diet®

Cancer: Fight It with the Blood Type Diet®

Cardiovascular Disease: Fight It with the Blood Type Diet®

Diabetes: Fight It with the Blood Type Diet®

Fatigue: Fight It with the Blood Type Diet®

DR. PETER J. D'ADAMO

WITH CATHERINE WHITNEY

Dr. Peter J. D'Adamo's

Eat Right for Your Type

Health Library

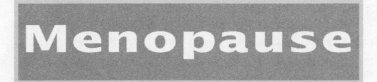

Menopause

Manage Its
Symptoms
with
the Blood
Type Diet®

BERKLEY BOOKS

NEW YORK

THE BERKLEY PUBLISHING GROUP
Published by the Penguin Group
Penguin Group (USA) Inc.
375 Hudson Street, New York, New York 10014, USA
Penguin Group (Canada), 90 Eglinton Avenue East, Suite 700, Toronto, Ontario M4P 2Y3, Canada
(a division of Pearson Penguin Canada Inc.)
Penguin Books Ltd., 80 Strand, London WC2R 0RL, England
Penguin Group Ireland, 25 St. Stephen's Green, Dublin 2, Ireland (a division of Penguin Books Ltd.)
Penguin Group (Australia), 250 Camberwell Road, Camberwell, Victoria 3124, Australia
(a division of Pearson Australia Group Pty. Ltd.)
Penguin Books India Pvt. Ltd., 11 Community Centre, Panchsheel Park, New Delhi—110 017, India
Penguin Group (NZ), Cnr. Airborne and Rosedale Roads, Albany, Auckland 1310, New Zealand
(a division of Pearson New Zealand Ltd.)
Penguin Books (South Africa) (Pty.) Ltd., 24 Sturdee Avenue, Rosebank, Johannesburg 2196,
South Africa

Penguin Books Ltd., Registered Offices: 80 Strand, London WC2R 0RL, England

While the author has made every effort to provide accurate telephone numbers and Internet addresses
at the time of publication, neither the publisher nor the author assumes any responsibility for errors,
or for changes that occur after publication. Further, publisher does not have any control over and does
not assume any responsibility for author or third-party websites or their content.

PRINTING HISTORY
G. P. Putnam's Sons hardcover edition / January 2006
Berkley trade paperback edition / December 2006

Berkley trade paperback ISBN: 0-425-21208-4

The Library of Congress has catalogued the G. P. Putnam's Sons hardcover edition as follows:

D'Adamo, Peter.
    Menopause: manage its symptoms with the blood type diet / Peter J. D'Adamo
    with Catherine Whitney.
        p.   cm.—(the eat right 4 your type health library)
    Includes index.
    ISBN 0-399-15253-9
    1. Menopause—Diet therapy.   2. Blood groups.   I. Whitney, Catherine.   II. Title.
    RG186.D25   2005   2005050993
    618.1'750654—dc22

PRINTED IN THE UNITED STATES OF AMERICA

10   9   8   7   6   5   4   3   2

DEDICATED TO THE PIONEERS IN
NATUROPATHY WHO SEEK SOLUTIONS
BEYOND THE PHARMACY

Acknowledgments

THIS BOOK OFFERS THE BEST THAT NATUROPATHIC MEDICINE and blood type science have to offer in helping women achieve well-being at midlife. It has been a collaborative process, and I want to express my deep thanks to the people who have been involved in its creation.

I am most grateful to Martha Mosko D'Adamo, not only my partner in life and in parenting but also my partner in bringing the valuable wisdom about blood type to the world. Martha daily provides love, support, insight, and inspiration to all of my endeavors.

Catherine Whitney, my writer, and her partner, Paul Krafin, are invaluable word masters who have once again captured exactly the right tone in tackling this complex topic.

My literary agent and friend, Janis Vallely, always takes time to listen and advise. Her quiet guidance and personal support make the work possible.

Special thanks to two friends and colleagues: Dr. Emily Kane, whose insight has been invaluable, and whose book, *Managing Menopause Naturally: Before, During, and Forever*, is an excellent guide for women; and Dr. Cathy Rogers, who continues to find ways to soothe and comfort women at every stage of life. I would also like to acknowledge Laura Mittman, N.D., of the Institute for Human Individuality, who has been such a big help in my efforts to educate other professionals about the value of the Blood Type Diet.

Amy Hertz, my former editor at Riverhead/Putnam, was the force behind the blood type books. Denise Silvestro continues to shepherd the work with dedication and skill. Catherine's agent, Jane Dystel, contributes her ideas and support.

As always, I am extremely grateful to the wonderful staff at Riverhead Books and Putnam. They have been tireless and enthusiastic, and their efforts have made it possible to continue bringing this important work to the market.

PETER J. D'ADAMO, N.D.

Contents

Appendices

Menopause

Manage Its Symptoms with the Blood Type Diet®

New Tools to Manage Menopausal Symptoms

THE BLOOD TYPE DIET CAN BENEFIT EVERYONE. YOU don't have to be sick to see the effects. But most of the people who come to my clinic or contact my Web site have a health problem they are trying to solve. They want to know how they can hone the general guidelines of the Blood Type Diet to address their unique circumstances. Dr. Peter J. D'Adamo's Eat Right 4 (for) Your Type Health Library has been introduced with these people in mind.

Menopause: Manage Its Symptoms with the Blood Type Diet allows you to take full advantage of the medicinal benefits of eating and living according to your blood type. If you think of the standard Blood Type Diet as the foundation, the guidelines in this book provide a more targeted overlay for women who want to maximize their health and well-being before, during, and after menopause. These dietary and lifestyle adaptations, individualized by blood type, help achieve those goals.

Here's what you'll find that's new:

- A health-enhancing category of blood type–specific food values, the **Super Beneficials,** emphasizing foods that have medicinal properties to minimize menopausal symptoms, strengthen immunity against disease, and improve metabolic health.
- A more detailed breakdown of the **Neutral** category to limit foods that are known to have less nutritional value. Foods designated **Neutral: Allowed Infrequently** should be minimized or avoided.
- Detailed supplement protocols for each blood type that are calibrated to support you at every stage. They include the **Basic Menopausal Support Protocol, Bone and Structural Support Protocol, Cardiovascular Fitness Protocol,** and **Skin Health and Vitality Protocol.**
- A **4 Week-Plan** for getting started that emphasizes what you can do right now to improve your condition and start feeling better immediately.
- Plus many strategies for success, checklists, and the answers to the questions most frequently asked about menopause at my clinic.

The chemistry of blood type continues to provide important clues to the biological and genetic mechanisms that control health and disease. Medical doctors and naturopaths throughout the world are increasingly applying the blood type principles in their practices, with remarkable results.

I urge you to talk to your physician about the benefits of incorporating individualized, blood type–specific diet, exercise, and lifestyle strategies into your current plan. I am confident that using the guidelines in this book will improve your state of being during menopause and beyond. Take the step now and use your blood type to your best advantage.

Why Blood
Type Matters

YOU ARE A BIOLOGICAL INDIVIDUAL.
Have you ever wondered why some people are constitutionally frail and susceptible to infection, while others seem naturally hardy? Why some people are able to lose weight on a particular diet, while others fail? Why some people age rapidly and show early signs of deterioration, while others are full of vitality into their later years?

We are all different. A single drop of your blood contains a biochemical signature as unique to you as your fingerprint. Many of the biochemical differences that make you an individual can be explained by your blood type.

Your blood type influences every facet of your physiology on a cellular level. It has everything to do with how you digest food, your ability to respond to stress, your mental state, the efficiency of your metabolic processes, and the strength of your immune system.

You can greatly improve your health, vitality, and emotional balance by knowing your blood type and by incorporating blood type–specific diet and lifestyle strategies into your health plan.

Be the biological individual you were meant to be!

PART I

Blood Type and Menopause: A Basic Primer

ONE

The Menopausal Woman

JUDGING BY THE CONCERNS EXPRESSED BY MY PATIENTS, most women view menopause as a state of diminished health. That's not surprising when you consider that pharmaceutical companies have worked so hard to "medicalize" this natural life transition.

It's amazing that in the twenty-first century, menopause is still steeped in so much myth and misinformation. When women at my clinic ask about menopause, they often do so fearfully, speaking in terms that imply it marks the end of their vibrancy, sexuality, and good health. It's a shame that these culturally embedded ideas about menopause date back more than a century, when the average life expectancy for women was fifty-two. Today, a healthy menopausal woman can expect to live a vital, active life for another thirty years or more. It's hardly an ending.

Nor is menopause a disease or sickness. We don't "treat" menopause at the clinic. We treat the *symptoms* of menopause. We also address the health problems that occur for many women at midlife—especially for those who are overweight, have high blood pressure, diabetes, smoke, or have metabolic disorders. For these women, the decline of ovarian function can exacerbate poor health conditions.

The main message I want you to take away from this book is that you are a biological individual. Your experience of menopause is unique. It is also holistic. If you are healthy, eat right for your type, exercise appropriately, and maintain a nontoxic (physically and mentally) environment, you won't automatically fall apart at menopause. If you have discomfort from menopausal symptoms, don't worry. They can be treated in a number of natural ways.

What Happens at Menopause?

THERE IS A TENDENCY to think of menopause as a single event—the dividing line between youth and age. In reality, it is a life process that begins before you're born.

Women are born with a finite number of eggs that eventually run out. At birth, a woman has close to a million eggs; by puberty, they have a mere 300,000. In the ten to fifteen years prior to menopause, the rate of loss begins to accelerate. Perimenopause is the term used to describe this time of transition between a woman's reproductive years and when menstruation ceases completely. Typically, perimenopause occurs between the ages of forty and fifty-one and may last anywhere from six months to ten years. During this time, hormone levels naturally fluctuate and decline, but they do not necessarily do so in an orderly manner. Shifts in hormone levels are a major contributor to that sense of physical, mental, and emotional imbalance that may characterize a woman's experience of menopause.

Eventually, estrogen levels decrease to the point that the lining of the uterus no longer builds up, and menstruation ceases. Menopause is defined as a cessation of periods for at least twelve months. After menopause, estrogen levels off at approximately 40 to 60 percent of its premenopausal levels, and progesterone falls close to zero. Although there are similarities in what happens hormonally, each woman's experience can be very different. Genetics may play a role in the timing, but diet and lifestyle have a substantial impact on your experience of menopause and on your health profile for the coming years.

Menopause:
A Highly Individual Experience

BECAUSE YOU ARE an individual with a unique environment, genetic makeup, and personal history, your experience of menopause may be very different than that of your mother, sisters, and female friends. Some women have virtually no symptoms beyond the end of their periods; some have only mild discomfort; others suffer greatly from a variety of symptoms. Here are the menopausal symptoms frequently reported:

Hot Flashes: The most common side effect of estrogen depletion, a hot flash is a sudden feeling of warmth throughout the upper part of the body, often accompanied by a reddening of the neck and face. Sweating occurs, followed by a cold, clammy sensation, chills, or shivers. Hot flashes can begin during perimenopause and last for years, but the average duration of the experience is about six months. They can vary in intensity: Some women report no problems, while others find them debilitating. Hot flashes have a diurnal rhythm with a peak intensity at night and a lesser intensity when the ambient temperature is low. They can be precipitated by stress, caffeine, alcohol, spicy foods, and skin-to-skin contact.

Vaginal Dryness and Infections: As estrogen levels decline, your genital area may become drier and thinner. This dryness can make sexual intercourse painful. Vaginal infections can become more common.

Weakened Bladder: The decrease in estrogen at menopause affects the bladder: The bladder wall and the supporting ligaments thin out. The bladder can "drop" and therefore lose its ability to fully empty during urination. The residual urine can cause bladder infections and incontinence. Some women find that urine leaks during exercise, sneezing, coughing, laughing, or running.

Lowered Libido: Some women report a flagging libido at menopause. However, your libido is not just controlled by sex hormones—it is also influenced by other factors, such as body image, fatigue, and the vaginal dryness that can be heightened by hormone depletion. Again, this is a highly individual experience. Some women report that the freedom from worrying about pregnancy actually improves their sex drives.

Sleep Problems: Some menopausal women report having trouble falling asleep or complain that they wake up frequently during the night. Night sweats and bladder problems may be partially to blame. Also, hormonal fluctuations can upset the natural sleep cycle.

Body and Skin Changes: Around the time of menopause, you may notice changes in your body, such as a thickening around the waist. A decline in collagen production can cause dry skin and hair. When you're young, your body produces plenty of collagen to renew your skin, but collagen production declines with age. In the five years after menopause, you can expect to lose up to 40 percent of your collagen. As a result, you'll begin to experience the dry skin, brown spots, and wrinkles that are the hallmarks of aging. While you can't halt the aging process, you can maintain fitness and skin health with dietary and lifestyle strategies for your blood type.

Midlife Risk Factors

IF YOU'RE THINKING about how to maximize your health in midlife and beyond, it's not just menopausal symptoms that should concern you. Your hormonal activity during this period affects your total physiology. Pay attention to the physiological risk factors that are associated with hormonal decline and aging, so you can fight them with the proper diet and exercise plan.

Bone Loss

Your body constantly builds new bone and removes older bone, but as you reach your middle years, declining hormone levels slow this process, resulting in lower bone density. After menopause, bone loss accelerates to an average of 1 to 2 percent a year. It can eventually lead to osteoporosis—a disease in which bones become fragile and more likely to break. You have a greater risk of osteoporosis if:

- You have a family history of osteoporosis
- You are Caucasian or Asian
- You have a small, thin frame
- You smoke
- You don't exercise regularly
- You take certain medications, such as cortisone or thyroid hormone
- You experienced early menopause, either naturally or through surgery

Weight-bearing exercise and bone-building nutrients can prevent osteoporosis—especially if you have paid attention to your bones long *before* menopause.

Heart Disease

Although younger women have a relatively low risk of heart disease, after menopause, a woman's risk of heart disease is almost the same as a man's. In fact, heart disease is the leading cause of death in women, leading to more deaths than lung or breast cancer. Hormonal fluctuations have an impact on your organ systems, including your heart and blood vessels. It's important to know your blood pressure, LDL (low-density lipoprotein) and HDL (high-density lipoprotein) cholesterol, triglycerides, and fasting blood glucose levels. You can lower your chance of heart disease by eating a healthy diet, not smoking, maintaining a healthy weight, and exercising regularly.

Insulin and Estrogen: A Synergistic Relationship

THE HORMONES INSULIN and estrogen have a synergistic relationship. If your insulin metabolism is out of balance, you won't be able to achieve a balance of your other hormones. A woman who is insulin resistant will not find relief from hot flashes or other menopausal symptoms with medications or herbal remedies, but she will certainly see her symptoms diminish if she controls her sugar levels. This is yet another example of how crucial diet is to maintaining health and well-being at menopause.

The Myth of Menopausal Depression

ONE OF THE BIGGEST myths of menopause is that menopausal women are depressed. Several major studies have found no evidence of this. Mood changes can be triggered by ill health, stress, and fatigue, but they are not necessarily a symptom of menopause. I wonder if the myth of menopausal depression arose from a cultural belief that women should be depressed by the loss of their fertility. My healthy, happy midlife patients tell me differently!

HRT: The Not-So-Magic Bullet

FOR MOST OF THE PAST thirty years, synthetic hormone replacement therapy in the form of popular formulations such as Premarin and Provera has been the gold standard of treatment. Women were told that taking these synthetic hormones would not only alleviate menopausal symptoms but also restore vitality, prevent bone loss, and protect them against heart disease.

Then, in 2002, the bubble burst. The Women's Health Initiative, a government-funded study of thousands of women who were prescribed Prempro (a combination estrogen-progesterone replacement therapy) found significant increases in blood clots, breast cancer, heart disease, and strokes. The trial was abruptly halted. Across the nation, doctors yanked their patients off HRT prescriptions.

For decades, HRT had been hailed for its benefits, which were believed to go far beyond minimizing menopausal symptoms. HRT was believed to protect against heart disease, improve bone strength, prevent urinary incontinence, improve libido, and even reduce wrinkles—a fountain of youth in a pill. But it turned out that HRT accomplished *none* of these miracles. The large-scale women's health trial, Heart and Estrogen/Progestin Replacement Study (HERS), conducted with women who already had heart disease, found that Premarin and Provera not only failed to protect against heart attacks but that the incidence of heart attacks actually *increased* in the first year of use. Meanwhile, the link between HRT and breast cancer, first established by the Harvard (University) Nurse's Health Study, was gaining credibility.

Many women were rightly feeling let down by a system that promised so much and offered so little. They had been taught to view menopause as a disease that must be treated, and now they had lost confidence in the treatment of choice. What to do?

If you discuss hormone replacement with your doctor, keep in mind that you are an individual, and you need to determine what's right for you. When it comes to managing menopause, one size does not fit all. Overall, I encourage my patients to use the Blood Type Diet to reduce the amount of medical intervention they need.

Is There a Male Menopause?

ALTHOUGH MEN DO NOT have the same cyclic hormonal nature as women, they do experience a decline in hormonal activity as they age. Male menopause (also called andropause) involves the hormonal, physiological, and chemical changes that generally occur between the ages of forty and fifty-five. These changes can affect all aspects of male physiology, not just sex drive. Low levels of testosterone in men can exert negative influences on both mood and mental abilities, including decline of memory and loss of youthful sexual function. Studies have shown that the sexual aging process results in organic impotence, ejaculatory and urinary problems, decreased sexual drive, dry skin, bone loss, and deterioration of the general physique.

KNOW YOUR HORMONES

Estrogen. Your body produces three estrogenic compounds: estradiol, estrone, and estriol. *Estradiol* is the most potent estrogen. In women, it's responsible for growth of the breast and reproductive epithelia, maturation of long bones, and development of the secondary sex characteristics. Estradiol is produced mainly by the ovaries with secondary production by the adrenal glands. Fat tissues also chip in by converting steroid precursors into estrogens. *Estrone* is produced primarily from androstenedione originating from the gonads or the adrenal cortex. After menopause, estrone levels increase, possibly due to increased conversion of androstenedione to estrone. *Estriol* is the weakest of the three estrogens, produced almost exclusively during pregnancy, and is the major estrogen produced in the normal human fetus. Estriol is thought to be less carcinogenic than estradiol and estrone and can be used at low doses and in topical preparations for the relief of menopausal symptoms.

Progesterone. A female hormone secreted by the corpus luteum after ovulation, which prepares the lining of the uterus for a fertilized egg. At menopause, progesterone levels decline to nearly zero. This decline can trigger many menopausal symptoms and contribute to metabolic imbalance and bone loss.

Testosterone. Although usually thought of as a male hormone, testosterone in smaller amounts is produced in the ovaries and adrenal glands of women. Testosterone builds muscle and bone and is responsible for maintaining libido.

DHEA (dehydroepiandrosterone). A steroid hormone made from cholesterol by the adrenal glands. DHEA enhances the activity of other hormones and contributes to energy levels, libido, and metabolic balance. It sharply declines after menopause.

Cortisol. This major stress hormone is an important regulator of energy metabolism. However, too much cortisol can cause systemic hormonal imbalances that tax your heart and immune system.

The Blood Type– Menopause Connection

THE ARRIVAL OF EACH IMPORTANT LIFE STAGE OFFERS YOU a new opportunity to rethink your wellness strategies. As you look ahead to the next thirty or so years, imagine yourself at the peak of health. Try to avoid judging yourself or your future based on what others say. While menopause itself is an inevitable passage for women, it's up to you to define your own limits and possibilities.

Your blood type can be a very useful tool in making that determination. Blood type is a key marker of individuality that gives you a picture of your strengths and weaknesses. You can use it to assess your risks for osteoporosis, heart disease, cancer, urinary incontinence, thyroid irregularities, and insulin resistance. These risk factors can often be ameliorated by adhering to the right diet and lifestyle recommendations for your blood type.

Blood Type:
Your Key to a Healthy Immune System

NATURE HAS ENDOWED our immune system with very sophisticated methods to determine if a substance in the body is foreign or not. One method involves looking for chemical markers, called antigens, which are found on the cells of our bodies and on most living things. Any substance could be an antigen; the only requirement is that it be unique enough to allow the immune system an opportunity to determine if it is "self" or "non-self." When an antigen encounters a harmful foreign intruder (such as a bacteria, virus, or parasite), it creates antibodies against it. These antibodies serve as an early warning system—the next time the foreign intruder is encountered, it will be attacked and destroyed.

Your blood type is expressed in every cell of your body, identified by its particular antigen. The same antigen-antibody dynamic that applies to your immune system applies to your blood type—which is why a transfusion with the wrong blood can be fatal. Blood Type O carries anti-A and anti-B antibodies, and rejects anything with an A-like or B-like antigen. Type A carries anti-B antibodies, and Type B carries anti-A antibodies. Only Type AB carries no anti–blood type antibodies, which is why Type AB individuals can receive blood transfusions from anybody.

Many substances, such as bacteria, viruses, parasites, and some foods, actually resemble foreign blood type antigens, and it is the job of your blood type antibodies to recognize these intruders and target them for removal. If your blood type antigen fails to produce antibodies to foreign substances, the result is a weakened immune system. That's an important consideration for you at midlife, because as we age, the amount of protective antibodies produced by our antigens declines, thus weakening our immune defenses. This decline can be delayed by maintaining a healthy immune system.

Blood Type Antigens and Antibodies

BLOOD TYPE	ANTIGENS	ANTIBODIES
O	None— or "zero" (fucose)	You produce antibodies to Blood Types A, B, and AB. You can only receive Type O blood, but you can donate blood to all types. Because of this, Type O is often referred to as the universal donor. However, your system considers all things in nature that are A-like or B-like foreign.
A	A	You produce antibodies to Blood Type B. You can receive blood from Blood Types O and A, but you consider all things in nature that are B-like foreign.
B	B	You produce antibodies to Blood Type A. You can receive blood from Blood Types O and B, but you consider all things in nature that are A-like foreign.
AB	A and B	Because both A and B antigens are present in your red blood cells, you don't carry antibodies for either. You can receive blood from Blood Types O, A, B, and AB. Because of this, Blood Type AB is often called the universal receiver.

Are You a Secretor or a Non-Secretor?

ANOTHER FACTOR relevant to your immune defenses is whether you are a secretor or a non-secretor. Although everyone carries a blood type antigen on their blood cells, about 80 percent of the population also secretes blood type antigens into body fluids, such as saliva, mucus, and sperm. These people are called secretors. The approximately 20 percent of the population that does not secrete blood type antigens into body fluids are called non-secretors. Being a secretor is independent of your ABO group: Thus, there are both Type O secretors and Type O non-secretors.

Since blood type antigens are crucial to immune defense, being unable to secrete them into body fluids can place non-secretors at a disadvantage. In general, non-secretors are more vulnerable to immune diseases than secretors, especially when the disease is provoked by an infectious organism.

What Does Diet Have to Do with It?

SIMPLY PUT, there are chemical reactions between your blood type antigen and the foods you eat. That's because the proteins in foods have antigens as well, and these antigens are similar to the blood type antigens. If you eat food that contains or resembles a foreign antigen, your blood type antigen will create antibodies to it, and it will be rejected by your system.

Lectins are proteins in foods that are capable of binding to antigens on blood cells, causing problems. The digestive impact of lectins is pervasive. They can interfere with the integrity of the digestive system, provoke inflammation, block digestive hormones, damage the intestinal lining, impair absorption, and interfere with protein digestion.

Many lectins are blood type–specific in that they show a clear preference for one kind of sugar over another and mechanically fit the antigen of one blood type or another. This blood type specificity results in their attaching to the antigen of a preferred blood type while leaving other blood type antigens completely undisturbed. Perhaps the most well-known effect of lectins occurs at the cellular level. They cause the sugars on the surface of one cell to cross-link with those of another, effectively causing the cells to stick together and agglutinate. Not all lectins cause agglutination. Many bacteria have lectinlike receptors that they use to attach to the cells of their host. Other lectins, called mitogens, cause a proliferation of certain cells of the immune system. But, in the most basic sense, lectins make things stick to other things.

Blood type–specific dietary lectins can wreak systemic havoc. They can interfere with protein absorption, prevent your digestive hormones from doing their job, damage your intestinal lining, promote insulin resistance, produce inflammatory conditions, and weaken your immune system. Most of my patients with chronic illnesses show the effects of some lectin activity. Knowing which lectins interact with your blood type and avoiding the foods that contain them can make a big difference to your overall health.

But it's not just a matter of avoiding harmful foods. Your blood type also recognizes foods that are beneficial—that support your unique chemical balance. The Blood Type Diet isn't only about saying no. It's also about saying yes!

Your Blood Type Profile at Menopause

MENOPAUSE AFFECTS every midlife woman regardless of her blood type, but knowing your blood type will help you negotiate this hormonal transition in the best of health.

If You Are Blood Type O . . .

Overall, if you are following the Blood Type Diet and a regular exercise program, you are less susceptible to some of the most common risk factors associated with hormone depletion, including osteoporosis and heart disease. Your risk factors for cancer are also lower than other blood types, making you a better candidate for hormone replacement, if you and your doctor decide to go that route.

Your greatest vulnerabilities at this time of life involve inflammatory diseases, metabolic syndrome, and poor thyroid regulation—most of which can be mediated by diet.

Your optimal diet is a high-protein, low-fat diet with limited grains and lots of fruits and vegetables. Wheat should be avoided altogether.

You may have heard that a high-protein diet can lead to excess calcium loss, which can be a concern for any midlife woman. However, this is not a danger for Blood Type O, since you have naturally high levels of intestinal alkaline phosphatase, an enzyme made by the intestine to split dietary fat and help assimilate calcium. Furthermore, the high-protein Type O Diet actually causes an increase in intestinal alkaline phosphatase.

If You Are Blood Type A . . .

You are most vulnerable to a range of conditions triggered by hormone depletion as well as hormone replacement. Your relatively high risk for cancer makes conventional hormone replacement especially tricky, as does your risk of blood clots. You should discuss alternatives with your doctor.

Your optimal diet is vegetarian with limited amounts of fish and fowl and greater amounts of healthy grains, beans, vegetables, and fruits. You should avoid red meat altogether and eat plenty of soy foods. Low levels of intestinal alkaline phosphatase and low hydrochloric acid make it difficult for you to digest meat and can make you vulnerable to osteoporosis. When you are not eating and living right for your type, you have a tendency to produce high levels of the stress hormone cortisol, which can place extra strain on your heart and exacerbate hormonal imbalance.

If You Are Blood Type B . . .

You have a generally good prognosis for most common effects of hormone depletion (osteoporosis, heart disease, cancer)—as long as you follow the Type B diet and exercise guidelines. Your optimal diet includes a balanced mix of meat, fish, dairy, fruits, and vegetables, with limited amounts of grains and beans. You should avoid chicken, corn, and wheat altogether, and you usually don't do well with soy foods.

Your greatest vulnerabilities at midlife are a tendency for slow-growing viral conditions, urinary tract infections, and insulin resistance—conditions usually mediated by diet. Like Type O, you have relatively high levels of intestinal alkaline phosphatase to aid protein digestion.

If You Are Blood Type AB . . .

You must negotiate carefully, as you have aspects of both A and B blood. Like Type A, you have a higher risk for cancer and blood clots—both factors in hormone replacement therapy. Low levels of intestinal alkaline phosphatase affect your bone health. Type AB has the highest incidence of osteoporosis of all the blood types.

Your optimal diet involves utilizing the best of A and B. That means a healthy mix of fish, soy, some meat and dairy, fruits and vegetables, and specific grains. Like Type B, you should avoid chicken and corn.

Is the Blood Type Diet the Fountain of Youth?

WE'VE ALL NOTICED that some people seem to "wear" their midlife years with a more youthful glow, and I'm not talking about the results of cosmetic surgery. Some of the variations are inherited, but much of the difference can be attributed to healthy living. If you are in good health, it will show in your skin and hair. As we mentioned earlier, the protective effects of your blood type antigen decline with age. Your task is to find ways to shore up your body's natural defenses. If renewed energy, stronger bones, good digestion, fewer colds and flu, and healthy skin comprise a fountain of youth, you can look forward to a maximum state of wellness as you embark upon the next stage of your life.

THREE

Addressing Menopause with Natural and Blood Type Therapies

MY FRIEND AND COLLEAGUE DR. EMILY KANE, N.D., L.A.c., strikes just the right tone in her book, *Managing Menopause Naturally Before, During, and Forever* (Basic Health Publications, 2004). She writes, "As a physician, I have consistently believed that hormone replacement therapy should be the last resort when treating women as they transition through menopause."

Dr. Kane points out that while some women can benefit from hormone replacement (preferably short-term, bioidentical), it should be used only as a last resort—after taking a full account of health, diet, and lifestyle issues that may be contributing to menopausal symptoms. I share this philosophy of treatment.

The problem with conventional medicine is that it tries to fit everybody into the same neat little box. Unfortunately, none of us is exactly the same. Every individual and their specific circumstances need to be taken into account. I urge you to find an ob-gyn who will listen to and work with you to find the perfect solution. In my experience, most doctors want to do what's best for their patients, so it's really a matter of communicating with them. You just need to find one who is willing to listen to you. You might also consider adding a licensed naturopathic physician to your health team. Consult my Web site (www.dadamo.com) for a list of naturopaths and MDs who use the Blood Type Diet in their practices.

The best way to approach perimenopause, menopause, and the postmenopausal years is by maximizing your health. That means eating right for your blood type, exercising regularly, reducing stress, and avoiding the chemical toxins in your environment. If you are functioning in peak condition and need extra support for menopausal symptoms, here are some general suggestions. Talk them over with your doctor.

Bioidentical Hormones

THE HORMONES USED in conventional preparations like Premarin are taken from the urine of pregnant mares. They are not natural to women. Bioidentical hormones made from plant sources like soy and wild yam, which are chemically identical—or bioidentical—to the estrogen, progesterone, and testosterone made in your body, are preferable.

But take note, just because they are natural doesn't mean that bioidentical hormones are necessarily safer for you. This is where you must assess what's right for you, weighing with your doctor the benefits and risks of hormone therapy and seeking the lowest dose for the shortest amount of time.

Phytoestrogens—A Natural Alternative

PHYTOESTROGENS ARE NATURALLY occurring plant compounds that act like estrogens in your body. However, phytoestrogens tend to have weaker effects than most estrogens, are not stored in the body, and can be easily broken down and eliminated. They don't pose the cancer risk found with estrogen replacement.

There is good evidence of a lower prevalence of breast cancer, heart disease, and hip fracture rates among women living in places like Southeast Asia, where diets are typically high in phytoestrogens. These women also tend to have fewer menopausal symptoms, such as hot flashes.

Phytoestrogens consist of more than 20 compounds and can be found in more than 300 plants, including herbs, grains, and fruits. The three main classes of dietary phytoestrogens are isoflavones, lignans, and coumestans:

- Isoflavones (genistein, diadzein, glycitein, and equol) are primarily found in soy beans and soy products, chickpeas, and other legumes.
- Lignans (enterolactone and enterodiol) are found in oil seeds (primarily flaxseed), cereal bran, legumes, and alcohol (beer and bourbon).
- Coumestans (coumestrol) can be found in alfalfa and clover.

Soy beans, the most potent phytoestrogen source, are made up of two primary components, soy protein and isoflavones, plant chemicals that have estrogenlike properties. The isoflavones genistein and diadzein in soy are thought to be responsible for relieving menopausal symptoms, like hot flashes. Soy protein in foods also lowers blood cholesterol levels, reducing the risk of heart disease for some women.

Before you start stocking up on soy products, however, let me make two very important points:

1. Stay away from the super soys! Many capsules heralded as super soys can do more harm than good. Eat your soy as food, don't pop it as pills.

2. If you have low thyroid function, be careful about your use of soy, as it can block thyroid receptors and worsen your condition.

How about Progesterone Creams?

I ADVISE YOU to be wary of topical progesterone, testosterone, and other hormonal creams sold in health-food stores and over the Internet. Many so-called "natural" progesterone creams do not contain substances that the human body can use as progesterone. Some products contain chemically synthesized progesterone, which is added to the plant extract in the cream. It isn't always possible for you to determine how much progesterone is being delivered through these creams.

Herbal Relief for
Menopausal Symptoms

HERBAL REMEDIES have been used for centuries to relieve menopausal symptoms and can serve as a helpful adjunct to your plan. You'll find blood type–specific suggestions in the Supplement Protocols section of the chapter devoted to your blood type.

Four Keys to Managing Menopausal
Symptoms with Blood Type Strategies

1. Eat Right for Your Blood Type

Most people are aware that deficiencies in essential nutrients can make them sick. For example, many dietary factors have been linked to lowered immunity. Failure to eat breakfast, irregular eating habits, low vegetable intake, inadequate protein, excessive wheat intake, reliance on highly processed foods, and high-fat diets have all been associated with weakened immune system defenses. Your diet is also crucial to proper metabolic balance and cardiovascular health.

Conventional nutritional wisdom has long held the view that a healthy diet is a balanced diet. Today that view is reflected in the USDA Recommended Daily Allowances and in the Food Pyramid, which represent a uniform approach to human nutrition. However, since all humans are not alike, these standards only apply in the most general way. They address food intake without factoring in variations in the ability to digest, metabolize, and utilize nutrients and efficiently eliminate wastes. These processes differ as people age, in conditions of chronic illness, and as a result of genetically inherited biochemical differences—such as those related to blood type.

Many foods contain components that can react directly with the blood type antigens, resulting in inflammation and the production of toxins. Other foods address susceptibilities and strengthen our bodies against these weaknesses, and when we consume them, we shift the odds in our favor.

Good digestion results from not only choosing the right foods for our bodies but also keeping our digestive systems tuned and balanced so that the interplay of all the important elements, such as digestive juices and hormones, is optimized for maximum nutrient absorption and regular elimination. As my father so aptly put it, "One man's food is another man's poison."

2. Exercise to Reduce Stress

The right kind of physical activity for your blood type can help you resist the bone, joint, and muscle deterioration associated with aging. Exercise has also been shown to boost mental acuity, improve mood, and help you recover from stress. Exercise also seems to be a great defense against the declines in immune function that occur with aging. In a few comparison studies of immune status between physically fit elderly individuals and young, not so physically fit sedentary controls, evidence suggests that habitual physical activity can enhance immune health. As a rule of thumb, there is no substitute for proper physical exercise if you wish to experience optimal health. The question is, what is the best exercise? That depends on your blood type. Your goal should be to reduce the overall load on your system, not to exhaust it. If you exert yourself beyond your level of tolerance, exercise can actually act as a stressor. Overexercise will spike cortisol levels for Blood Type A individuals, furthering exhaustion. On the other hand, Blood Type O thrives on vigorous aerobic exercise, while Blood Types B and AB fall somewhere in between.

3. Clean Out the Toxins

There are many causes of the accumulated cellular damage that becomes noticeable with aging. Among these are the oxidative processes and related free radical damage that result from UV sunlight, smog, toxins, cigarette smoke, X-rays, drugs, and other stressors. As we age, our bodies experience increased wear and tear; at the same time, the energy needed for cell repair and renewal becomes increasingly diminished and the antioxidant enzymes less available.

Foods rich in ribonucleic acids (RNA) such as sardines, salmon, tuna, and legumes help improve cellular energy. Foods rich in antioxidants and other phytochemicals such as fruits, vegetables, and green tea help protect against oxidative damage and free radical attack on all body cells including the skin. The oral intake of supplements—particularly the antioxidants vitamins E and C and the mineral selenium, and vitamin A, the "skin vitamin," together with supplements of RNA and B vitamins (for coenzymes) and the minerals zinc, copper, and manganese—provide even more intensive protection against damaging free radicals.

The accumulation of toxins can create damage in your gastrointestinal tract. By balancing intestinal flora and improving digestive acid production, it is possible to restore gastrointestinal health and reduce the inflammatory responses of the digestive system, giving it more strength to fight off the disease state. Friendly intestinal bacteria protect your cells, improve immune function, and have a positive effect on your ability to fully utilize the nutrients in the foods you eat. Blood type antigens orchestrate the proper balance of friendly bacteria in your system. Consumption of probiotics—lactic acid bacteria, or food cultured or fermented with these friendly microorganisms—does extend life in animal experiments and does dramatically reduce a wide range of intestinal metabolites, including indoles, polyamines, cresols, nitrates/nitrites, and carcinogens that we now know are counterproductive to good health. It is even more beneficial if you consume friendly bacteria specific to your blood type, since bacteria show favoritism for the sugars of one blood type over another.

4. Use Supplementation According to Your Blood Type

Blood type–specific supplement protocols are calibrated to provide extra ammunition to help you control the symptoms of menopause. Refer to your blood type section for details.

ARE YOU READY TO START? Find your blood type section, and we'll get you on the right diet for your type to manage menopausal symptoms.

PART II

Individualized Blood Type Plans

FOUR

Blood Type

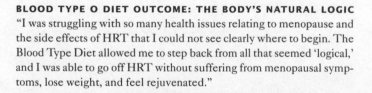

BLOOD TYPE O DIET OUTCOME: THE BODY'S NATURAL LOGIC
"I was struggling with so many health issues relating to menopause and the side effects of HRT that I could not see clearly where to begin. The Blood Type Diet allowed me to step back from all that seemed 'logical,' and I was able to go off HRT without suffering from menopausal symptoms, lose weight, and feel rejuvenated."

BLOOD TYPE O DIET OUTCOME: RENEWAL!
"For about five years, before and during menopause, I found myself losing my natural high energy and good health. I was experiencing continual fatigue and muscle aches, along with sore throats, colds, and hot flashes. Within two weeks of going on the Type O Diet and sticking to it rigidly, my energy came back, I was able to sleep through the night, I could exercise without resultant pain, and my hot flashes were reduced to a mild warmth from time to time. When I do eat foods that are detrimental to me, I almost always feel the negative results (grogginess, lack of energy, foggy brain, headaches, hot flashes). One of my goals was to get through menopause without taking estrogen replacement, and the Blood Type Diet has helped me to achieve that."

Self-reported outcomes from the Blood Type Diet Web site (www.dadamo.com).

Blood Type O: The Foods

THE BLOOD TYPE O Menopause Diet is specifically adapted to provide the maximum nutritional support to protect your health and fight the symptoms of menopause. A new category, **Super Beneficial** highlights powerful disease-fighting foods for Blood Type O. The **Neutral** category has also been adjusted to de-emphasize foods that are less advantageous for you. Foods designated **Neutral: Allowed Infrequently** should be minimized or avoided entirely.

Your secretor status can influence your ability to fully digest and metabolize certain foods, so various adjustments in the values are made for non-secretors. If you do not know your secretor type, the odds are that you can safely use the "secretor" values, since the majority of the population (approximately 80 percent) are secretors. However, I urge you to get tested, since the variations are important for non-secretors who want to maximize the effectiveness of the Blood Type Diet.

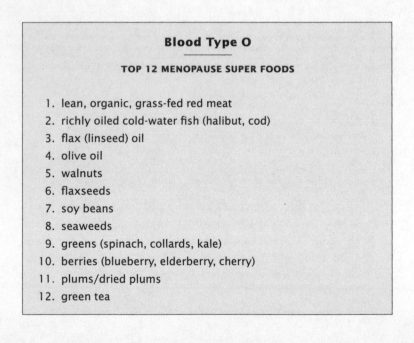

Blood Type O

TOP 12 MENOPAUSE SUPER FOODS

1. lean, organic, grass-fed red meat
2. richly oiled cold-water fish (halibut, cod)
3. flax (linseed) oil
4. olive oil
5. walnuts
6. flaxseeds
7. soy beans
8. seaweeds
9. greens (spinach, collards, kale)
10. berries (blueberry, elderberry, cherry)
11. plums/dried plums
12. green tea

The food charts are divided into three sections. The top of the chart suggests the average portion size and quantity per week or day, according to secretor status. These recommendations do *not* apply to the category **Neutral: Allowed Infrequently**; those foods should be eaten rarely, if at all. The charts also indicate differences in frequency for some foods based on ethnic heritage. It has been my experience that this factor has an impact upon the individual's ability to fully digest certain foods. For the purposes of blood type food choices, persons of Hispanic heritage should follow the guidelines for Caucasians, and American Native peoples should follow the guidelines for Asians.

The middle section of the chart gives the food values. The bottom section lists variants based on secretor status.

For your convenience, we have included a number of product names (Ezekiel 4:9 bread, Worcestershire sauce, etc.). However, keep in mind that commercial formulations vary among brands and regions. Even though a product may be listed as acceptable for you, always check its ingredients. Some products contain **Avoid** ingredients for your blood type. Of course, you may choose to make your own version of commercial products, such as bread and mayonnaise, using ingredients that suit your blood type. There are hundreds of delicious recipes for every blood type available on our Web site (www.dadamo.com) and in the book *Cook Right 4 Your Type: The Practical Kitchen Companion to Eat Right 4 Your Type.*

Meat/Poultry

Protein, in the form of lean, organic meat, is critical for Blood Type O and is the key to digestive health and immune function. In particular, grass-fed beef is high in omega-3 fatty acids and the essential fatty acid conjugated linoleic acid (CLA), which improves metabolic activity and protects the heart. Make sure your chicken is organic and hormone-free to minimize unhealthy estrogen activity. Choose only the best quality (preferably free-range) chemical-, antibiotic-, and pesticide-free low-fat meats and poultry. Grass-fed cattle and buffalo are far superior to grain-fed.

BLOOD TYPE O: MEAT/POULTRY			
Portion: 4–6 oz (men); 2–5 oz (women and children)			
	African	Caucasian	Asian
Secretor	6–9	6–9	6–9
Non-Secretor	7–12	7–12	7–11
		Times per week	

SUPER BENEFICIAL	BENEFICIAL	NEUTRAL: Allowed Frequently	NEUTRAL: Allowed Infrequently	AVOID
Beef	Heart (calf)	Chicken		All commercially
Buffalo	Liver (calf)	Cornish hen		processed
Lamb	Mutton	Duck		meats
	Sweetbreads	Goat		Bacon/ham/pork
	Veal	Goose		Quail
	Venison	Grouse		Turtle
		Guinea hen		
		Horse		
		Ostrich		
		Partridge		
		Pheasant		
		Rabbit		
		Squab		
		Squirrel		
		Turkey		

Special Variants: *Non-Secretor:* BENEFICIAL: ostrich, partridge, pheasant, rabbit, squab; NEUTRAL (Allowed Frequently): lamb, liver (calf), quail, turtle.

Fish/Seafood

Fish and seafood represent a secondary source of high-quality protein for Blood Type O. In particular, richly oiled cold-water fish like cod, halibut, red snapper, and trout are SUPER BENEFICIAL for Blood Type O. These fish contain beneficial omega-3 fatty acids, such as docosahexaenoic acid (DHA) and eicosapentaenoic acid (EPA), which can help improve thyroid function, counter inflammatory conditions, and regulate metabolism.

BLOOD TYPE O: FISH/SEAFOOD			
Portion: 4–6 oz (men); 2–5 oz (women and children)			
	African	Caucasian	Asian
Secretor	2–4	3–5	2–5
Non-Secretor	2–5	4–5	4–5
		Times per week	

SUPER BENEFICIAL	BENEFICIAL	NEUTRAL: Allowed Frequently	NEUTRAL: Allowed Infrequently	AVOID
Cod	Bass (all)	Anchovy	Eel	Abalone
Halibut	Perch (all)	Beluga	Flounder	Barracuda
Red snapper	Pike	Bluefish	Gray sole	Catfish
Trout (rainbow)	Shad	Bullhead	Grouper	Conch
	Sole (except gray)	Butterfish	Whitefish	Frog
	Sturgeon	Carp		Herring (pickled/ smoked)
	Swordfish	Caviar (sturgeon)		Muskellunge
	Tilefish	Chub		Octopus
	Yellowtail	Clam		Pollock
		Crab		Salmon (smoked)
		Croaker		
		Cusk		
		Drum		

SUPER BENEFICIAL	BENEFICIAL	NEUTRAL: Allowed Frequently	NEUTRAL: Allowed Infrequently	AVOID
		Haddock		Salmon roe
		Hake		Squid (calamari)
		Halfmoon fish		
		Harvest fish		
		Herring (fresh)		
		Lobster		
		Mackerel		
		Mahimahi		
		Monkfish		
		Mullet		
		Mussel		
		Opaleye		
		Orange roughy		
		Oysters		
		Parrot fish		
		Pickerel		
		Pompano		
		Porgy		
		Rosefish		
		Sailfish		
		Salmon (caught, not farm raised)		
		Sardine		
		Scallops		
		Scrod		
		Shark		
		Shrimp		

SUPER BENEFICIAL	BENEFICIAL	NEUTRAL: Allowed Frequently	NEUTRAL: Allowed Infrequently	AVOID
		Smelt		
		Snail (*Helix pomatia*/ escargot)		
		Sucker		
		Sunfish		
		Tilapia		
		Trout (brook/ sea)		
		Tuna		
		Weakfish		
		Whiting		

Special Variants: *Non-Secretor:* BENEFICIAL: hake, herring (fresh), mackerel, sardine; NEUTRAL (Allowed Frequently): bass, catfish, halibut, red snapper, salmon roe; AVOID: anchovy, crab, mussel.

Dairy/Eggs

Most dairy foods should be avoided by Blood Type O. They are poorly digested and metabolized, resulting in indigestion, weight gain, inflammation, and fatigue. Ghee (clarified butter) is one exception because it's a good source of butyrate, which supports Blood Type O intestinal health. Eggs can be consumed in moderation. Do your best to find eggs and dairy products that are both hormone-free and organic.

BLOOD TYPE O: EGGS			
Portion: 1 egg			
	African	Caucasian	Asian
Secretor	1–4	3–6	3–4
Non-Secretor	2–5	3–6	3–4
	Times per week		

BLOOD TYPE O: MILK AND YOGURT			
Portion: 4–6 oz (men); 2–5 oz (women and children)			
	African	Caucasian	Asian
Secretor	0–1	0–3	0–2
Non-Secretor	0	0–2	0–3
		Times per week	

BLOOD TYPE O: CHEESE			
Portion: 3 oz (men); 2 oz (women and children)			
	African	Caucasian	Asian
Secretor	0–1	0–2	0–1
Non-Secretor	0	0–1	0
		Times per week	

SUPER BENEFICIAL	BENEFICIAL	NEUTRAL: Allowed Frequently	NEUTRAL: Allowed Infrequently	AVOID
	Ghee (clarified butter)	Egg (chicken/ duck)	Butter	American cheese
			Farmer cheese	Blue cheese
			Feta	Brie
			Goat cheese	Buttermilk
			Mozzarella	Camembert
				Casein
				Cheddar
				Colby
				Cottage cheese
				Cream cheese
				Edam
				Egg (goose/ quail)
				Emmenthal
				Gouda

SUPER BENEFICIAL	BENEFICIAL	NEUTRAL: Allowed Frequently	NEUTRAL: Allowed Infrequently	AVOID
				Gruyère
				Half-and-half
				Ice cream
				Jarlsberg
				Kefir
				Milk (cow/goat)
				Monterey Jack
				Muenster
				Neufchâtel
				Paneer
				Parmesan
				Provolone
				Quark
				Ricotta
				Sherbet
				Sour cream
				String cheese
				Swiss cheese
				Whey
				Yogurt

Special Variants: *Non-Secretor:* NEUTRAL (Allowed Frequently): Egg (goose/quail); AVOID: farmer cheese, feta, goat cheese, mozzarella.

Oils

Olive oil, a monounsaturated oil, is SUPER BENEFICIAL for Blood Type O. Constituents in olive oil, such as flavonoids, squalenes, and polyphenols, act as powerful antioxidants. It should be used as the primary cooking oil. Flax (linseed) oil is high in phytoestrogen lignans, which regulate hormonal activity and reduce menopausal symptoms. Be aware that some oils are high in omega-6 fatty acids, which can stimulate an inflammatory response. These include corn, cottonseed, peanut, and safflower oils. Secretors have a bit of an edge over non-secretors in digesting oils and probably benefit a bit more from their consumption.

BLOOD TYPE O: OILS			
Portion: 1 tblsp			
	African	Caucasian	Asian
Secretor	3–8	4–8	5–8
Non-Secretor	1–7	3–5	3–6
		Times per week	

SUPER BENEFICIAL	BENEFICIAL	NEUTRAL: Allowed Frequently	NEUTRAL: Allowed Infrequently	AVOID
Flax (linseed) Olive		Almond Black currant seed Borage seed Cod liver Sesame Walnut	Canola	Avocado Castor Coconut Corn Cottonseed Evening primrose Peanut Safflower Soy Sunflower Wheat germ
Special Variants: *Non-Secretor:* BENEFICIAL: almond, walnut; NEUTRAL (Allowed Frequently): coconut, flax (linseed); AVOID: borage seed, canola, cod liver.				

Nuts/Seeds

Overall, Blood Type O should limit intake of nuts and seeds in favor of high-quality animal protein. However, raw flax (linseed) are helpful for a strong immune system, providing beneficial omega-3 fatty acids. Raw flaxseeds also contain beneficial lignans that help regulate hormonal activity. Walnuts are also SUPER BENEFICIAL. They are one of the best plant sources of omega-3 fatty acids.

BLOOD TYPE O: NUTS/SEEDS			
Portion: Whole (handful); Nut Butters (2 tblsp)			
	African	Caucasian	Asian
Secretor	2–5	2–5	2–4
Non-Secretor	5–7	5–7	5–7
		Times per week	

SUPER BENEFICIAL	BENEFICIAL	NEUTRAL: Allowed Frequently	NEUTRAL: Allowed Infrequently	AVOID
Flax (linseed) Walnut (black/ English)	Pumpkin seed	Almond Almond butter Almond cheese Almond milk Butternut Filbert (hazel- nut) Hickory Macadamia Pecan	Safflower seed Sesame butter (tahini) Sesame seed	Beechnut Brazil nut Cashew Chestnut Lychee Peanut Peanut butter Pistachio Poppy seed Sunflower butter Sunflower seed

SUPER BENEFICIAL	BENEFICIAL	NEUTRAL: Allowed Frequently	NEUTRAL: Allowed Infrequently	AVOID
		Pignolia (pine nut)		

Special Variants: *Non-Secretor:* NEUTRAL (Allowed Frequently): flax (linseed); AVOID: almond cheese, almond milk, safflower seed.

Beans and Legumes

Essentially carnivores when it comes to protein requirements, Blood Type Os should minimize consumption of beans and legumes. Given the choice, get your protein from animal foods. An exception for menopausal women may be soy beans. They contain isoflavones that help minimize symptoms, build up bone, and protect the heart.

BLOOD TYPE O: BEANS AND LEGUMES			
Portion: 1 cup (cooked)			
	African	Caucasian	Asian
Secretor	1–3	1–3	2–4
Non-Secretor	0–2	0–3	2–4
			Times per week

SUPER BENEFICIAL	BENEFICIAL	NEUTRAL: Allowed Frequently	NEUTRAL: Allowed Infrequently	AVOID
Fava (broad) bean	Adzuki bean Bean (green/ snap/ string) Black-eyed pea	Black bean Cannellini bean Garbanzo (chickpea)	Soy milk	Copper bean Kidney bean Lentil (all) Navy bean Pinto bean

SUPER BENEFICIAL	BENEFICIAL	NEUTRAL: Allowed Frequently	NEUTRAL: Allowed Infrequently	AVOID
	Northern bean	Jicama bean		Tamarind bean
		Lima bean		
		Mung bean/ sprouts		
		Pea (green/ pod/ snow)		
		Soy bean		
		Soy cheese		
		Soy, miso		
		Soy, tempeh		
		Soy, tofu		
		White bean		

Special Variants: *Non-Secretor:* NEUTRAL (Allowed Frequently): adzuki bean, black-eyed pea, lentil (all), pinto bean. AVOID: fava (broad) bean, garbanzo (chickpea), soy (all).

Grains and Starches

Blood Type O does poorly on corn, wheat, sorghum, barley, and many of their by-products (sweeteners, etc.). In particular, the lectin in wheat produces gut inflammation and is the primary cause of celiac disease. Wheat is also a leading factor in Blood Type O's susceptibility to autoimmune thyroid disease, inflammation, and insulin resistance. The exceptions are sprouted seed breads, such as Essene and Ezekiel 4:9, usually found in the freezer section of your health-food store. Non-secretors have even greater wheat sensitivity. Non-secretors should avoid oats as well.

BLOOD TYPE O: GRAINS AND STARCHES			
Portion: ½ cup dry (grains or pastas); 1 muffin; 2 slices of bread			
	African	**Caucasian**	**Asian**
Secretor	1–6	1–6	1–6
Non-Secretor	0–3	0–3	0–3
			Times per week

SUPER BENEFICIAL	BENEFICIAL	NEUTRAL: Allowed Frequently	NEUTRAL: Allowed Infrequently	AVOID
	Essene bread (manna)	Amaranth Ezekiel 4:9 bread Kamut Quinoa Spelt (whole) Spelt flour/ products Tapioca Teff 100% sprouted grain products (except Essene)	Buckwheat Millet Oat bran Oat flour Oatmeal Rice (whole) Rice (wild) Rice cake Rice flour Rice milk Rye (whole) Rye flour/ products Soba noodles (100% buck-wheat) Soy flour/ products	Barley Cornmeal Couscous Grits Popcorn Sorghum Wheat (re-fined/un-bleached) Wheat (semolina) Wheat (white flour) Wheat (whole) Wheat bran Wheat germ

Special Variants: *Non-Secretor:* AVOID: buckwheat, oat (all), soba noodles (100% buckwheat), soy flour/products, spelt (whole), spelt flour/products, tapioca.

Vegetables

Vegetables provide a rich source of antioxidants and fiber, and the right choices can help Blood Type O balance immune functions. Seaweeds are effective in blocking lectin activity and are a good source of iodine, which helps Type Os improve thyroid function. Broccoli contains the phytochemical indole-3-carbinol, which converts strong estrogens to less carcinogenic estrogens. Beets are natural estrogen sources. Collards, kale, and spinach are rich in antioxidants and good sources of calcium.

Vegetables in the so-called nightshade family—white potatoes, bell peppers, eggplant, and tomatoes—should be avoided. They are pro-inflammatory and can interfere with thyroid function.

An item's value also applies to its juice, unless otherwise noted.

BLOOD TYPE O: VEGETABLES			
Portion: 1 cup, prepared (cooked or raw)			
	African	Caucasian	Asian
Secretor Super/ Beneficials	Unlimited	Unlimited	Unlimited
Secretor Neutrals	2–5	2–5	2–5
Non-Secretor Super/Beneficials	Unlimited	Unlimited	Unlimited
Non-Secretor Neutrals	2–3	2–3	2–3
	Times per day		

SUPER BENEFICIAL	BENEFICIAL	NEUTRAL: Allowed Frequently	NEUTRAL: Allowed Infrequently	AVOID
Beet greens	Artichoke	Arugula	Brussels sprouts	Alfalfa sprouts
Broccoli	Chicory	Asparagus	Cabbage	Aloe
Collards	Escarole	Asparagus pea		Cauliflower

SUPER BENEFICIAL	BENEFICIAL	NEUTRAL: Allowed Frequently	NEUTRAL: Allowed Infrequently	AVOID
Kale Seaweeds Spinach	Horse- radish Kohlrabi Lettuce (Romaine) Mushroom (abalone/ enoki/ maitake/ oyster/ porto- bello/ straw/ tree ear) Okra Onion (all) Parsnip Potato (sweet) Pumpkin Swiss chard Turnip	Bamboo shoot Beet Bok choy Carrot Celeriac Celery Chili pepper Daikon radish Endive Fennel Fiddlehead fern Garlic Lettuce (except Romaine) Poi Radicchio Radish/ sprouts Rappini (broccoli rabe) Rutabaga Scallion Shallot Squash Water chestnut	Olive (Greek/ green/ Spanish) Yam	Corn Cucumber Eggplant Leek Mushroom (shiitake/ silver dollar) Mustard greens Olive (black) Peppers (all) Potato Tomato

SUPER BENEFICIAL	BENEFICIAL	NEUTRAL: Allowed Frequently	NEUTRAL: Allowed Infrequently	AVOID
		Watercress Zucchini		

Special Variants: *Non-Secretor:* BENEFICIAL: carrot, fiddlehead fern, garlic; NEUTRAL (Allowed Frequently): lettuce (Romaine), mushroom (except shiitake), mustard greens, parsnip, potato (sweet), turnip; AVOID: Brussels sprouts, cabbage, eggplant, olive (all), poi.

Fruits and Fruit Juices

Blood Type O should consume lots of fruits rich in antioxidants, vitamins, and fiber. Blueberries, cherries, and elderberries contain bioflavonoids, a potent phytoestrogen. Plums contain phytonutrients that reduce free radical damage. Bananas are excellent sources of potassium, promoting healthy circulation and lowering blood pressure.

SUPER BENEFICIAL are blueberries, cherries, and elderberries, which lower the production of toxins. Several citrus fruits, such as kiwi and oranges, contain O-reactive lectins, so are best avoided if you are suffering from irritable bowel syndrome.

An item's value also applies to its juices, unless otherwise noted.

BLOOD TYPE O: FRUITS AND FRUIT JUICES			
Portion: 1 cup			
	African	Caucasian	Asian
Secretor	2–4	3–5	3–5
Non-Secretor	1–3	1–3	1–3
	Times per day		

SUPER BENEFICIAL	BENEFICIAL	NEUTRAL: Allowed Frequently	NEUTRAL: Allowed Infrequently	AVOID
Blueberry	Banana	Boysen-	Apple	Asian pear
Cherry	Fig (fresh/	berry	Apricot	Avocado
Elderberry	dried)	Breadfruit	Currant	Bitter melon
(dark	Guava	Canang	Date	Blackberry
blue/	Mango	melon	Grape (all)	Cantaloupe
purple)	Pineapple	Casaba	Quince	Coconut
	Plum	melon	Raisin	Honeydew
	Prune	Christmas	Star fruit	Kiwi
		melon	(caram-	Orange
		Cranberry	bola)	Plantain
		Crenshaw	Strawberry	Tangerine
		melon		
		Dewberry		
		Goose-		
		berry		
		Grapefruit		
		Kumquat		
		Lemon		
		Lime		
		Logan-		
		berry		
		Mulberry		
		Muskmelon		
		Nectarine		
		Papaya		
		Peach		
		Pear		
		Persian		
		melon		
		Persimmon		
		Pome-		
		granate		

SUPER BENEFICIAL	BENEFICIAL	NEUTRAL: Allowed Frequently	NEUTRAL: Allowed Infrequently	AVOID
		Prickly pear		
		Raspberry		
		Sago palm		
		Spanish melon		
		Water- melon		
		Young- berry		

Special Variants: *Non-Secretor:* BENEFICIAL: avocado, pomegranate, prickly pear; NEUTRAL (Allowed Frequently): elderberry (dark blue/purple); AVOID: apple, apricot, date, strawberry.

Spices/Condiments/Sweeteners

Many spices have medicinal properties. Turmeric improves liver function. Garlic improves immune health and is anti-inflammatory. Cayenne pepper is also anti-inflammatory, although you might want to limit intake if you have hot flashes. Many common food additives, such as guar gum and carrageenan, enhance the effects of lectins found in other foods and should be avoided. Use caution when using prepared condiments, as they often contain wheat.

SUPER BENEFICIAL	BENEFICIAL	NEUTRAL: Allowed Frequently	NEUTRAL: Allowed Infrequently	AVOID
Garlic	Carob	Agar	Apple pectin	Aspartame
Parsley	Fenugreek	Allspice	Arrowroot	Caper
Turmeric	Ginger	Almond extract		Carrageenan

SUPER BENEFICIAL	BENEFICIAL	NEUTRAL: Allowed Frequently	NEUTRAL: Allowed Infrequently	AVOID
	Horse-radish	Anise	Barley malt	Cornstarch
	Pepper (cayenne)	Basil	Chocolate	Corn syrup
		Bay leaf	Honey	Dextrose
		Bergamot	Ketchup	Fructose
		Caraway	Maple syrup	Guarana
		Cardamom	Molasses	Gums (acacia/ Arabic/ guar)
		Chervil	Molasses (black-strap)	Invert sugar
		Chili powder	Rice syrup	Juniper
		Chive	Senna	Mace
		Cilantro (coriander leaf)	Soy sauce	Maltodex-trin
		Cinnamon	Sucanat	MSG
		Clove	Sugar (brown/ white)	Nutmeg
		Coriander		Pepper (black/ white)
		Cream of tartar		Vinegar (except apple cider)
		Cumin		Worcester-shire sauce
		Dill		
		Gelatin, plain		
		Lecithin		
		Licorice root*		
		Marjoram		
		Mayonnaise		
		Mint (all)		
		Mustard (dry)		
		Oregano		
		Paprika		

SUPER BENEFICIAL	BENEFICIAL	NEUTRAL: Allowed Frequently	NEUTRAL: Allowed Infrequently	AVOID
		Pepper (pepper-corn/red flakes)		
		Rosemary		
		Saffron		
		Sage		
		Savory		
		Sea salt		
		Stevia		
		Tamari (wheat-free)		
		Tamarind		
		Tarragon		
		Thyme		
		Vanilla		
		Vegetable glycerine		
		Vinegar (apple cider)		
		Winter-green		
		Yeast (baker's/brewer's)		

Special Variants: *Non-Secretor:* BENEFICIAL: basil, bay leaf, licorice root,* oregano, saffron, tarragon, yeast (brewer's); NEUTRAL (Allowed Frequently): carob, MSG, nutmeg, turmeric; AVOID: agar, barley malt, cinnamon, honey, maple syrup, mayonnaise, rice syrup, sage, soy sauce, stevia, sucanat, sugar (brown/white), tamari (wheat-free), vanilla, vinegar (apple cider).

*Do not use if you have high blood pressure.

Herbal Teas

Herbal teas can provide medicinal benefits and are excellent replacements for caffeinated drinks such as coffee, cola, and black tea. SUPER BENEFICIAL herbal teas for Blood Type O include dandelion, which aids liver function; sarsaparilla, which is an anti-inflammatory and binds endotoxin; and valerian, which is an antistress remedy and sleep aid.

SUPER BENEFICIAL	BENEFICIAL	NEUTRAL: Allowed Frequently	NEUTRAL: Allowed Infrequently	AVOID
Dandelion	Chickweed	Catnip	Senna	Alfalfa
Sarsaparilla	Fenugreek	Chamomile		Aloe
Valerian	Ginger	Dong quai		Burdock
	Hops	Elder		Coltsfoot
	Linden	Ginseng		Corn silk
	Mulberry	Hawthorn		Echinacea
	Peppermint	Horehound		Gentian
	Rosehip	Licorice		Goldenseal
	Slippery elm	Mullein		Red clover
		Raspberry leaf		Rhubarb
		Skullcap		Shepherd's purse
		Spearmint		St. John's wort
		Vervain		Strawberry leaf
		White birch		Yellow dock
		White oak bark		
		Yarrow		

Special Variants: None.

Miscellaneous Beverages

Blood Type Os with menopausal symptoms should avoid coffee, which can exacerbate hot flashes. Soda can contribute to bone loss. Green tea should be part of every Blood Type O's health plan. It contains polyphenols, which block the production of intestinal toxins. Avoid or limit alcohol to an occasional glass of red wine. Try to eliminate coffee by slowly weaning yourself off and replacing it with green tea. The tea has less caffeine but more positive benefits.

SUPER BENEFICIAL	BENEFICIAL	NEUTRAL: Allowed Frequently	NEUTRAL: Allowed Infrequently	AVOID
Tea (green)	Seltzer Soda (club)		Wine (red)	Beer Coffee (reg/ decaf) Liquor Soda (cola/ diet/misc.) Tea, black (reg/ decaf) Wine (white)

Special Variants: *Non-Secretor:* BENEFICIAL: Wine (red).

Supplements

THE BLOOD TYPE O DIET offers abundant quantities of important nutrients, such as protein and iron. It is important to get as many nutrients as possible from fresh foods, and use supplements only to fill in the minor deficiencies in your diet. The following supplement protocols are designed for Blood Type O women to support health during and after menopause.

Note: If you are being treated for a medical condition, consult your doctor before taking any supplements.

Blood Type O:
Basic Menopausal Support Protocol

Use this protocol for 6 weeks.		
SUPPLEMENT	**ACTION**	**DOSAGE**
High-quality multiple vitamin complex (preferably blood type–specific)	Supports general health	As directed
Chaste berry (*Vitex agnus-castus*)	Acts upon the pituitary gland to increase progesterone production	400 mg standardized, 1 capsule, twice daily
Vervain (*Verbena officialis*)	Acts as a nerve tonic, sedative, antispasmodic, and hypertensive agent	As tea, 1–2 cups daily
Dandelion (*Taraxacum officinale*)	Supports digestive health; used to treat constipation, edema, heartburn, and liver ailments	1 capsule, twice daily

Blood Type O:
Bone and Structural Support Protocol

Use this protocol for 6 weeks.		
SUPPLEMENT	**ACTION**	**DOSAGE**
High-quality multiple vitamin complex (preferably blood type–specific)	Supports general health	As directed

SUPPLEMENT	ACTION	DOSAGE
Horsetail (*Equisetum arvense*)	Helps alleviate menopausal symptoms; protects against brittle bones	500 mg, 1 capsule, twice daily
Manganese	Essential mineral for skin, bone, and cartilage formation; protects against osteoporosis	5 mg, 1 capsule daily
Vitamin A	Antioxidant immune support; necessary for bone health	10,000 IU, 1 capsule daily
Boron	Helps maintain healthy bones; enhances the metabolism of calcium, magnesium, copper, phosphorus, and vitamin D	1 mg, 1 capsule daily
Calcium (from sea plants)	Maintains bone strength	1,000 mg daily

Blood Type O: Cardiovascular Fitness Protocol

Use this protocol for 6 weeks

SUPPLEMENT	ACTION	DOSAGE
Arjuna myrobalan (*Terminalia arjuna*) 2% arjunolic acid	Promotes cardiac health	250 mg, twice daily
Coleus (*Coleus forskohlii*)	Enhances intracellular energy production; reduces blood pressure	Standardized extract: 125 mg, twice daily
L-carnitine	Enhances intracellular energy production; reduces blood pressure	50 mg, twice daily

SUPPLEMENT	ACTION	DOSAGE
Guggul gum (*Commiphora mukul*)	Provides vascular support; lowers cholesterol	Standardized for 25 mg guggulsterones of types E and Z: 1 capsule, once or twice daily
Bladderwrack (*Fucus vesiculosus*)	Improves metabolic function; regulates thyroid activity	200 mg, twice daily

Blood Type O: Skin Health and Vitality Protocol

Use this protocol for 4 weeks.		
SUPPLEMENT	ACTION	DOSAGE
Probiotic (preferably blood type–specific)	Improves intestinal health; promotes detoxification	As directed
Vitamin A	Antioxidant; reduces oxidative damage	10,000 IU, 1 capsule daily
Biotin	Antifungal; promotes skin health	2 mg, 2 capsules daily
Pantothenic acid (vitamin B_5)	Balances adrenal activity and reduces the effects of stress; reduces allergic reactions	500 mg, twice daily
(Non-secretors) Tea tree (*Leptospermum sp*) oil lotion (5%)	Treatment of acne, eczema, and fungal infections	Apply topically, twice daily, as needed

---

GENERAL RECOMMENDATIONS USABLE BY ALL GROUPS

Topical treatment with witch hazel (*Hamamelis virginiana*) as needed

Topical treatment with marigold juice (*Calendula officinalis*) as needed

Zinc, 15 mg: 1 capsule, twice daily
Niacinamide cream (4%): apply topically, twice daily

The Exercise Component

REGULAR EXERCISE is one of the best things you can do for your heart, bones, and overall fitness at menopause. Blood Type O benefits tremendously from brisk exercise that taxes the cardiovascular and musculoskeletal systems. Build a balanced routine of both aerobic and strength-training activities from the following chart. If you are not accustomed to exercising, or you are suffering from a chronic condition, start slowly and do as much as you can, striving to increase your time and endurance as you gain flexibility and strength.

EXERCISE	DURATION	FREQUENCY
Aerobics	40–60 minutes	3–4 x week
Weight training	30–45 minutes	3–4 x week
Running	40–45 minutes	3–4 x week
Calesthenics	30–45 minutes	3 x week
Treadmill	30 minutes	3 x week
Kickboxing	30–45 minutes	3 x week
Cycling	30 minutes	3 x week
Contact sports	60 minutes	2–3 x week
In-line/roller skating	30 minutes	2–3 x week

3 Steps to Effective Exercise

1. Warm up with stretching and flexibility moves before you start your aerobic exercise.
2. To achieve maximum cardiovascular benefits, work toward an elevated heart rate that is about 70 percent of your capacity. Once you reach the elevated rate, continue exercising to

maintain that rate for twenty to thirty minutes. To calculate your maximum heart rate and performance level:
- Subtract your age from 220.
- Multiply the difference by .70 (or .60 if you are over age sixty). This is the high end of your performance.
- Multiply the remainder by .50. This is the low end of your performance.

3. Finish each aerobic session with at least a five-minute cooldown of stretching and relaxation moves.

Getting Started: The First Month

IF YOU ARE NEW to the Blood Type Diet, the following guidelines will introduce you to the Blood Type O regimen over a period of one month. Follow these recommendations as closely as possible, using a notebook to record your personal experiences with the diet. In addition to factors that are measurable in laboratory tests, take the time to note changes in your energy levels, sleep patterns, digestion, and overall well-being.

I advise that you keep a daily journal of your symptoms, the times they occur, and the circumstances. This will help you better manage them. If you are experiencing perimenopause, keep a record of your cycles and the changes you notice.

Blood Type O Diet Checklist
for the Menopausal Woman

Eat small to moderate portions of high-quality, lean,   ☐
organic, grass-fed meat several times a week for strength.

Include regular portions of richly oiled cold-water fish.   ☐

Consume little or no dairy foods.   ☐

Eliminate wheat and wheat-based products from your diet. ☐

Limit your intake of beans principally to those that are BENEFICIAL. ☐

Eat lots of BENEFICIAL fruits and vegetables. ☐

Avoid stimulants found in caffeine (coffee, colas, etc.). ☐

Avoid coffee, but drink green tea every day. ☐

Exercise daily. Do as much as you comfortably can. Start with modest goals but try to do a bit more each day. ☐

Week 1

Blood Type Diet and Supplements

- Eliminate your most harmful AVOID foods—wheat and dairy. These foods are the primary triggers for many health problems that afflict Blood Type O.
- Include your most important BENEFICIAL foods on a regular schedule throughout the week. For example, have lean red meat 5 times, and omega-3-rich fish 3 to 4 times, with lots of BENEFICIAL vegetables and fruit.
- Incorporate at least 1 SUPER BENEFICIAL food into your daily diet. For example, eat a snack of walnuts and cherries, or add seaweed to your salad.
- If you're a coffee drinker, begin to wean yourself by cutting your daily consumption in half. Substitute green tea.

Exercise Regimen

- Plan to exercise at least 4 days this week, for 45 minutes each day.
  2 days: aerobic activity
  2 days: weights
- Use your journal to detail the time, activity, distance, and amount of weight lifted. Note the number of repetitions for each exercise.

▪ WEEK 1 SUCCESS STRATEGY ▪
Cool Down the Hot Flashes

Here are some natural ways to keep your hot flashes in check:

- Wear layered clothing so you can remove items if you feel overheated during the day.

- Avoid caffeine and alcohol; they can trigger flashes in some women.
- Minimize your use of hot spices like cayenne pepper.
- Certain medications, such as those prescribed to lower blood pressure, can bring on flashes. If this is a problem, ask your doctor to prescribe a different formula.
- A tepid shower can help bring down body temperature.

Week 2

Blood Type Diet and Supplements

- Begin to eliminate the next level of AVOID foods—corn, potatoes, beans, and legumes.
- Eat at least 2 BENEFICIAL animal proteins every day, choosing from the meat, poultry, and seafood lists.
- Initially, it is best to avoid foods listed as NEUTRAL: Allowed Infrequently.
- Continue to incorporate SUPER BENEFICIAL foods into your daily diet.
- If you're a coffee drinker, continue to cut your coffee intake, substituting green tea.
- Manage your mealtimes to aid proper digestion. Avoid eating on the run. Make your meals relaxing, sit-down affairs. Eat slowly and chew thoroughly to encourage digestive secretions and better digestion.

Exercise Regimen

- Continue to exercise at least 4 days this week, for 45 minutes each day.
  2 days: aerobic activity
  2 days: weights
- If your work is sedentary, get in the habit of taking a couple of "movement" breaks during the day. Walk around the block or take the stairs instead of the elevator.

■ WEEK 2 SUCCESS STRATEGY ■
Regulate Your Thyroid Activity

Type Os have a special susceptibility to thyroid problems, caused by either an overproduction (hyperthyroidism) or underproduction (hypothyroidism) of the thyroid hormone thyroxine. To regulate your thyroid activity, follow the Type O Diet and adhere to the following protocol for a period of four weeks:

- Dandelion (*Taraxacum officinale*): 250 mg, 1 capsule, twice daily
- Guggul gum (*Commiphora mukul*): Standardized for 25 mg guggulsterones of types E and Z: 1 capsule, once or twice daily
- Selenium: 50–75 mcg daily
- Lectin-blocking formula ("Deflect") specific for Type O: 2 capsules with meals
- Green tea: 1–3 cups daily
- Diet: Incorporate iodine-rich foods, especially seaweeds and safe saltwater fish, into your diet

Week 3

Blood Type Diet and Supplements

- When you plan your meals for week 3, choose BENEFICIAL or SUPER BENEFICIAL foods to replace NEUTRAL foods whenever possible. For example, choose lean, organic beef or buffalo over chicken, or blueberries over an apple.
- Eliminate all remaining AVOID foods.
- Liberally incorporate SUPER BENEFICIAL foods into your daily diet.
- Completely wean yourself from coffee, substituting green or herbal tea.

Exercise Regimen

- Continue to exercise at least 4 days this week, for 45 minutes each day.
  2 days: aerobic activity
  2 days: weights

- **WEEK 3 SUCCESS STRATEGY** -
You're Never Too Old to Start Exercising

Often I will treat a woman in her forties or fifties who has never been an exerciser and is intimidated by the prospect. Invariably, these women feel as if it's too late for them to start.

Maybe you used to be active but haven't exercised regularly

in a long time. Before you begin, get a checkup from your doctor to rule out conditions that may impede physical activity. It may help to find a walking buddy or join a light aerobics class. As baby boomers age, more health clubs are designing programs for the fifty-plus. A great resource is the AARP Web site (www.AARP.org), which offers strategies for age-appropriate exercise.

Week 4

Blood Type Diet and Supplements

- Continue at the week 3 level, focusing on BENEFICIAL and SUPER BENEFI-CIAL foods.
- Evaluate the first 4 weeks and make adjustments.

Exercise Regimen

- Continue at the week 3 level.
- Review your progress, noting in your journal improvements in strength, flexibility, and overall energy. Determine which exercise regimen has worked for you, including time of day, setting, and activity level.

■ WEEK 4 SUCCESS STRATEGY ■
Clean Up Your Internal Environment

Getting rid of toxins that inhibit metabolic activity and increase vulnerability to infection (such as *Candida albicans*) is job one for Type O. The right blend of beneficial bacteria in the gut will help eliminate the interior atmosphere that encourages fungal growth. Start with a probiotic supplement, preferably blood type specific. Your blood type antigens are prominent in your digestive tract, and, if you are a secretor, they are also prominent in the mucus that lines your digestive tract. Because of this, many of the bacteria in your digestive tract use your blood type as a preferred food supply. In fact, blood group specificity is common among intestinal bacteria with almost half of strains tested showing some blood type A, B, or O specificity. For more information about blood type–specific probiotics, go to the Web site www.dadamo.com.

FIVE

Blood Type

A

BLOOD TYPE A DIET OUTCOME: A SUCCESS STORY

"By walking two to three miles every day and sticking to the Blood Type A Diet, I lost thirteen pounds in six weeks or so, and was never really hungry. Also my menopausal symptoms have lowered to almost nothing. Hot flashes are only slight or not at all. My skin and hair look better and I am in better moods. I can honestly say that I have not felt this good in quite some time. I thought I felt good before, but of course feel better now. I never go hungry on the Blood Type Diet either. Also my food cravings have confirmed what my body needs, which has corresponded to the Blood Type Diet."

BLOOD TYPE A DIET OUTCOME: NEW AND IMPROVED

"I started the Blood Type Diet and gave up wheat, dairy, red meat, sugar, and alcohol. I also stopped taking three of my doctor prescribed meds (hormone, cholesterol, antidepressant). I began receiving acupuncture to help me with my cravings, especially my addiction to alcohol. When I began the diet, I weighed 142 pounds (five feet three inches and age forty-five). In six weeks I am down to 128. I have a lot more energy, feel much more relaxed, and my digestion/elimination, sleeping, and overall well-being have improved. Before I began the program, I felt as if I was headed toward having a heart attack (seriously). My lifestyle and eating habits were horrible. Now I've cleaned up my act and feel like a new person. My family cannot believe the change! Thank you so much for helping me become a 'new and improved' person."

Self-reported outcomes from the Blood Type Diet Web site (www.dadamo.com).

Blood Type A: The Foods

THE BLOOD TYPE A Menopause Diet is specifically adapted to provide the maximum nutritional support to protect your health and fight the symptoms of menopause. A new category, **Super Beneficial**, highlights powerful disease-fighting foods for Blood Type A. The **Neutral** category has also been adjusted to de-emphasize foods that are less advantageous for you. Foods designated **Neutral: Allowed Infrequently** should be minimized or avoided entirely.

Your secretor status can influence your ability to fully digest and metabolize certain foods, so various adjustments in the values are made for non-secretors. If you do not know your secretor type, the odds are that you can safely use the "secretor" values, since the majority of the population (approximately 80 percent) are secretors. However, I urge you to get tested, since the variations are important for non-secretors who want to maximize the effectiveness of the Blood Type Diet.

The food charts are divided into three sections. The top of the chart suggests the average portion size and quantity per week or day, according to secretor status. These recommendations do *not* apply to the category **Neutral: Allowed Infrequently**; those foods should be eaten rarely, if at all. The charts also indicate differences in frequency for some foods, based on ethnic heritage. It has been my experience that this factor has an impact upon the individual's ability to fully digest certain foods. For the purposes of blood type food choices, persons of Hispanic heritage should follow the guidelines for Caucasians, and American Native peoples should follow the guidelines for Asians.

Blood Type A

TOP 12 MENOPAUSE SUPER FOODS

1. soy-based foods
2. richly oiled cold-water fish (salmon, sardines)

3. olive oil
4. flax (linseed) oil
5. walnuts
6. flaxseeds
7. dark leafy greens (spinach, kale, Swiss chard)
8. broccoli
9. alfalfa
10. berries (blueberry, cherry, elderberry)
11. garlic
12. green tea

The middle section of the chart gives the food values. The bottom section lists variants based on secretor status.

For your convenience, we have included a number of product names (Ezekiel 4:9 bread, Worcestershire sauce, etc.). However, keep in mind that commercial formulations vary among brands and regions. Even though a product may be listed as acceptable for you, always check its ingredients. Some products contain **Avoid** ingredients for your blood type. Of course, you may choose to make your own version of commercial products, such as bread and mayonnaise, using ingredients that suit your blood type. There are hundreds of delicious recipes for every blood type available on our Web site (www.dadamo.com) and in the book *Cook Right 4 Your Type: The Practical Kitchen Companion to Eat Right 4 Your Type.*

Meat/Poultry

Blood Type A lacks some of the enzymes and stomach acids needed to effectively digest animal protein. When you overconsume meat, the undigested by-products can foster a toxic intestinal environment. For this reason, Blood Type A should derive most of its protein from non-meat sources. Non-secretors have a small advantage over secretors in the ability to digest animal protein but should still derive most of their protein from foods other than meat. Choose only the best-quality (preferably free-range) chemical-, antibiotic-, and pesticide-free low-fat meats and poultry.

BLOOD TYPE A: MEAT/POULTRY

Portion: 4–6 oz (men); 2–5 oz (women and children)

	African	Caucasian	Asian
Secretor	0–2	0–3	0–3
Non-Secretor	2–5	2–4	2–3
	Times per week		

SUPER BENEFICIAL	BENEFICIAL	NEUTRAL: Allowed Frequently	NEUTRAL: Allowed Infrequently	AVOID
		Chicken		All commercially processed meats
		Cornish hen		Bacon/ham/pork
		Grouse		Beef
		Guinea hen		Buffalo
		Ostrich		Duck
		Squab		Goat
		Turkey		Goose
				Heart (beef)
				Horse
				Lamb
				Liver (calf)
				Mutton
				Partridge
				Pheasant
				Quail
				Rabbit

SUPER BENEFICIAL	BENEFICIAL	NEUTRAL: Allowed Frequently	NEUTRAL: Allowed Infrequently	AVOID
				Squirrel
				Sweet-breads
				Turtle
				Veal
				Venison

Special Variants: *Non-Secretor*: BENEFICIAL: turkey; NEUTRAL (Allowed Frequently): duck, goat, goose, lamb, mutton, partridge, pheasant, quail, rabbit, turtle.

Fish/Seafood

Fish and seafood represent a nutritious source of protein for Blood Type A. SUPER BENEFICIAL are the richly oiled cold-water fish, such as cod, mackerel, salmon, sardines, and trout. These are high in omega-3 fatty acids, such as docosahexaenoic acid (DHA) and eicosapentaenoic acid (EPA), which can help to balance immune function and reduce inflammation. The *Helix pomatia* snail (escargot) contains a lectin SUPER BENEFICIAL for Type A's immune system.

BLOOD TYPE A: FISH/SEAFOOD			
Portion: 4–6 oz (men); 2–5 oz (women and children)			
	African	Caucasian	Asian
Secretor	1–3	1–3	1–3
Non-Secretor	2–5	2–5	2–4
	Times per week		

SUPER BENEFICIAL	BENEFICIAL	NEUTRAL: Allowed Frequently	NEUTRAL: Allowed Infrequently	AVOID
Cod	Carp	Abalone		Anchovy
Mackerel	Monkfish	Bass (sea)		Barracuda
Salmon (caught, not farm raised)	Perch (silver/ yellow)	Bullhead		Bass (bluegill/ striped)
	Pickerel	Butterfish		
		Chub		Beluga
Sardine	Pollock	Croaker		Bluefish
Snail (*Helix pomatia/ escargot*)	Red snapper	Cusk		Catfish
		Drum		Caviar (sturgeon)
	Trout (sea)	Halfmoon fish		
Trout (rainbow)	Whitefish	Mahimahi		Clam
	Whiting	Mullet		Conch
		Muskel- lunge		Crab
				Crayfish
		Orange roughy		Eel
		Parrot fish		Flounder
		Perch (white)		Frog
				Gray sole
		Pike		Grouper
		Pompano		Haddock
		Porgy		Hake
		Rosefish		Halibut
		Sailfish		Harvest fish
		Salmon roe		Herring (fresh/ pickled/ smoked)
		Scrod		
		Shark		
		Smelt		
		Sturgeon		Lobster
		Sucker		Mussel
		Sunfish		Octopus
		Swordfish		Opaleye
		Tilapia		Oysters

SUPER BENEFICIAL	BENEFICIAL	NEUTRAL: Allowed Frequently	NEUTRAL: Allowed Infrequently	AVOID
		Trout (brook)		Salmon (smoked)
		Tuna		Scallops
		Weakfish		Scup
		Yellowtail		Shad
				Shrimp
				Sole
				Squid (calamari)
				Tilefish

Special Variants: *Non-Secretor:* BENEFICIAL: chub, cusk, drum, halfmoon fish, harvest fish, mullet, muskellunge, perch (white), pompano, rosefish, sailfish, sucker, swordfish, trout (brook); NEUTRAL (Allowed Frequently): anchovy, bass (bluegill), beluga, bluefish, caviar (sturgeon), flounder, frog, gray sole, grouper, haddock, hake, halibut, herring (fresh), mussel, octopus, opaleye, scallops, scup, shad, tilefish.

Dairy/Eggs

Dairy foods should mostly be avoided by Blood Type A, especially those prone to frequent colds or excess mucus production. Exceptions are cultured dairy products and eggs, in moderation. Do your best to find eggs and dairy products that are both hormone-free and organic.

BLOOD TYPE A: EGGS			
Portion: 1 egg			
	African	Caucasian	Asian
Secretor	1–3	1–3	1–3
Non-Secretor	2–3	2–5	2–4
	Times per week		

BLOOD TYPE A: MILK AND YOGURT			
Portion: 4–6 oz (men); 2–5 oz (women and children)			
	African	Caucasian	Asian
Secretor	0–1	1–3	0–3
Non-Secretor	0–1	1–2	0–2
		Times per week	

BLOOD TYPE A: CHEESE			
Portion: 3 oz (men); 2 oz (women and children)			
	African	Caucasian	Asian
Secretor	0–2	1–3	0–2
Non-Secretor	0	0–1	0–1
		Times per week	

SUPER BENEFICIAL	BENEFICIAL	NEUTRAL: Allowed Frequently	NEUTRAL: Allowed Infrequently	AVOID
		Egg (chicken/ duck/ goose/ quail) Farmer cheese Ghee (clarified butter) Kefir Mozzarella	Feta Goat cheese Milk (goat) Sour cream	American cheese Blue cheese Brie Butter Buttermilk Camembert Casein Cheddar Colby Cottage cheese

SUPER BENEFICIAL	BENEFICIAL	NEUTRAL: Allowed Frequently	NEUTRAL: Allowed Infrequently	AVOID
		Paneer		Cream cheese
		Ricotta		Edam
		Yogurt		Emmenthal
				Gouda
				Gruyère
				Half-and-half
				Ice cream
				Jarlsberg
				Milk (cow)
				Monterey Jack
				Muenster
				Neufchâtel
				Parmesan
				Provolone
				Sherbet
				Swiss cheese
				Whey

Special Variants: *Non-Secretor:* NEUTRAL (Allowed Frequently): cottage cheese, whey; AVOID: milk (goat), sour cream.

Oils

Olive oil, a monounsaturated fat, is SUPER BENEFICIAL for Blood Type A. Constituents in olive oil are powerful antioxidants. It should be used as a primary cooking oil. Flax (linseed) oil is high in phytoestrogen lignans, which regulate hormonal activity and reduce menopausal symptoms.

Be aware that some oils are high in omega-6 fatty acids, which can stimulate the inflammatory response. These include corn, cottonseed, and peanut oils.

BLOOD TYPE A: OILS			
Portion: 1 tblsp			
	African	**Caucasian**	**Asian**
Secretor	5–8	5–8	5–8
Non-Secretor	3–7	3–7	3–6
	Times per week		

SUPER BENEFICIAL	BENEFICIAL	NEUTRAL: Allowed Frequently	NEUTRAL: Allowed Infrequently	AVOID
Flax (linseed) Olive	Black currant seed Walnut	Almond Avocado Borage seed Cod liver Evening primrose Safflower Sesame Soy Sunflower Wheat germ	Canola	Castor Coconut Corn Cottonseed Peanut

Special Variants: *Non-Secretor:* BENEFICIAL: cod liver, sesame; NEUTRAL (Allowed Frequently): peanut; AVOID: safflower.

Nuts/Seeds

Nuts and seeds can serve as an important secondary source of protein for Blood Type A. Laboratory research has identified at least five natural phytochemicals in nuts that regulate the immune system and act as antioxidants. SUPER BENEFICIAL for Blood Type A are flax (linseed) and walnuts, which are high in omega-3 fatty acids. Flax (linseed) also contain beneficial lignans that help regulate hormonal activity.

BLOOD TYPE A: NUTS/SEEDS			
Portion: Whole (handful); Nut Butters (2 tblsp)			
	African	Caucasian	Asian
Secretor	4–7	4–7	4–7
Non-Secretor	5–7	5–7	5–7
	Times per week		

SUPER BENEFICIAL	BENEFICIAL	NEUTRAL: Allowed Frequently	NEUTRAL: Allowed Infrequently	AVOID
Flax (linseed) Walnut (black/ English)	Peanut Peanut butter Pumpkin seed	Almond Almond butter Almond cheese Almond milk Beechnut Butternut Chestnut Filbert (hazelnut) Hickory nut	Safflower seed Sesame butter (tahini) Sesame seed	Brazil nut Cashew Pistachio

SUPER BENEFICIAL	BENEFICIAL	NEUTRAL: Allowed Frequently	NEUTRAL: Allowed Infrequently	AVOID
		Lychee		
		Macadamia nut		
		Pecan		
		Pignolia (pine nut)		
		Poppy seed		
		Sunflower butter		
		Sunflower seed		

Special Variants: *Non-Secretor:* AVOID: safflower seed, sunflower butter, sunflower seed.

Beans and Legumes

Blood Type A thrives on vegetable proteins found in many beans and legumes. In particular, soy beans are BENEFICIAL for menopausal women. They contain isoflavones that help minimize symptoms, build bone, and protect against cancer. Soy isoflavones also inhibit the enzyme aromatase (which converts steroids to estrogens) and so help build lean muscle mass. Try to avoid the "supersoy" high isoflavone products, and get the benefits of soy from true food sources.

BLOOD TYPE A: BEANS AND LEGUMES			
Portion: 1 cup (cooked)			
	African	Caucasian	Asian
Secretor	5–7	5–7	5–7
Non-Secretor	3–5	3–5	3–5
		Times per week	

SUPER BENEFICIAL	BENEFICIAL	NEUTRAL: Allowed Frequently	NEUTRAL: Allowed Infrequently	AVOID
Soy bean Soy cheese Soy milk Soy, miso Soy, tempeh Soy, tofu	Adzuki bean Bean (green/snap/string) Black bean Black-eyed pea Fava (broad) bean Lentil (all) Pinto bean	Cannellini bean Jicama bean Mung bean/sprouts Northern bean Pea (green/pod/snow) White bean		Copper bean Garbanzo (chickpea) Kidney bean Lima bean Navy bean Tamarind bean

Special Variants: *Non-Secretor:* NEUTRAL (Allowed Frequently): adzuki bean, bean (green/snap/string), black bean, black-eyed pea, copper bean, fava (broad) bean, kidney bean, navy bean, soy bean and products.

Grains and Starches

Blood Type A benefits from a moderate consumption of grains. Amaranth is a good source of phytoestrogens. If you suffer from frequent colds and infections or have a serious illness, limit or avoid wheat and corn. This is especially important for non-secretors.

BLOOD TYPE A: GRAINS AND STARCHES			
Portion: ½ cup dry (grains or pastas); 1 muffin; 2 slices of bread			
	African	Caucasian	Asian
Secretor	7–10	7–9	7–10
Non-Secretor	5–7	5–7	5–7
	Times per week		

SUPER BENEFICIAL	BENEFICIAL	NEUTRAL: Allowed Frequently	NEUTRAL: Allowed Infrequently	AVOID
Amaranth Soy flour/ products	Buckwheat Essene bread (manna) Ezekiel 4:9 bread Oat bran Oat flour Oatmeal Rice (whole) Rice bran Rye (whole) Soba noodles (100% buck- wheat)	Barley Kamut Quinoa Rice (wild) Rice cake Rice flour/ products Rice milk Rye flour/ products Sorghum Spelt (whole) Spelt flour/ products Wheat (re- fined/un- bleached) Wheat (semo- lina) Wheat (white flour) 100% sprouted grain products (except Essene, Ezekiel 4:9)	Cornmeal Couscous Grits Millet Popcorn Tapioca Wheat (whole)	Teff Wheat bran Wheat germ

Special Variants: *Non-Secretor:* NEUTRAL (Allowed Frequently): buckwheat, Ezekiel 4:9 bread, oat (all), soba noodles (100% buckwheat), soy flour/products, teff; AVOID: cornmeal, couscous, grits, popcorn, wheat (all).

Vegetables

Antioxidant-rich vegetables, such as broccoli, spinach, and dark greens protect against free radical damage. Broccoli contains the phytochemical indole-3-carbinol, which converts strong estrogens to less carcinogenic estrogens. Spinach and kale are also good sources of calcium. Alfalfa is a good source of phytoestrogens. Artichokes can help the liver detoxify more efficiently.

Tomatoes contain a lectin that reacts with the saliva and digestive juices of Blood Type A secretors, although it does not appear to react with non-secretors. Yams are typically high in the amino acid phenylalanine, which inactivates intestinal alkaline phosphatase (already quite low in Blood Type A) and should be minimized or avoided completely.

An item's value also applies to its juices, unless otherwise noted.

BLOOD TYPE A: VEGETABLES			
Portion: 1 cup, prepared (cooked or raw)			
	African	Caucasian	Asian
Secretor Super/ Beneficials	Unlimited	Unlimited	Unlimited
Secretor Neutrals	2–5	2–5	2–5
Non-Secretor Super/Beneficials	Unlimited	Unlimited	Unlimited
Non-Secretor Neutrals	2–3	2–3	2–3
			Times per day

SUPER BENEFICIAL	BENEFICIAL	NEUTRAL: Allowed Frequently	NEUTRAL: Allowed Infrequently	AVOID
Alfalfa sprouts	Aloe	Arugula	Corn	Cabbage
Artichoke	Beet	Asparagus	Olive (green)	Eggplant
Broccoli	Beet greens	Asparagus pea	Pickle (in brine)	Mushroom (shiitake)
	Carrot			

SUPER BENEFICIAL	BENEFICIAL	NEUTRAL: Allowed Frequently	NEUTRAL: Allowed Infrequently	AVOID
Kale	Celery	Bamboo shoot	Squash (all)	Olive (black/ Greek/ Spanish)
Spinach	Chicory	Beet		Peppers (all)
Swiss chard	Collards	Bok choy		Pickle (in vinegar)
	Escarole	Brussels sprouts		Potato
	Garlic	Cabbage (juice)*		Potato (sweet)
	Horse-radish	Cauli-flower		Rhubarb
	Kohlrabi	Celeriac		Tomato
	Leek	Cucumber		Yam
	Lettuce (Romaine)	Daikon radish		Yucca
	Mushroom (maitake/ silver dollar)	Endive		
	Okra	Fennel		
	Onion (all)	Fiddlehead fern		
	Parsnip	Lettuce (except Romaine)		
	Pumpkin	Mung bean/ sprouts		
	Rappini (broccoli rabe)	Mushroom (abalone/ enoki/ oyster/ porto-bello/ straw/ tree ear)		
	Turnip	Mustard greens		
		Oyster plant		

SUPER BENEFICIAL	BENEFICIAL	NEUTRAL: Allowed Frequently	NEUTRAL: Allowed Infrequently	AVOID
		Poi		
		Radicchio		
		Radish/ sprouts		
		Rutabaga		
		Scallion		
		Seaweeds		
		Shallot		
		Taro		
		Water chestnut		
		Watercress		
		Zucchini		

Special Variants: *Non-Secretor:* NEUTRAL (Allowed Frequently): alfalfa sprouts, aloe, carrot, celery, eggplant, garlic, horseradish, lettuce (Romaine), mushroom (maitake/shiitake), peppers (all), potato (sweet), rappini (broccoli rabe), tomato; AVOID: agar, cabbage (juice), mushroom (silver dollar), pickle (in brine).

*To obtain the benefits of cabbage juice, it must be consumed within one minute of juicing.

Fruits and Fruit Juices

Eat lots of fruits rich in antioxidants, vitamins, and fiber. In particular, berries are super antioxidants and anti-aging catalysts. Blueberries, cherries, and elderberries contain bioflavonoids, a potent phytoestrogen. Plums and prunes contain antioxidants that decrease free radical damage (as do most purple and blue fruits). They are also good iron sources for Type A.

An item's value also applies to its juice, unless otherwise noted.

BLOOD TYPE A: FRUITS AND FRUIT JUICES			
Portion: 1 cup			
	African	**Caucasian**	**Asian**
Secretor	2–4	3–4	3–4
Non-Secretor	2–3	2–3	2–3
		Times per day	

SUPER BENEFICIAL	BENEFICIAL	NEUTRAL: Allowed Frequently	NEUTRAL: Allowed Infrequently	AVOID
Blackberry	Apricot	Apple	Currant	Banana
Blueberry	Boysen-	Asian pear	Date	Bitter melon
Cherry	berry	Avocado	Grape (all)	Coconut
Elderberry	Cranberry	Breadfruit	Pomegranate	Honeydew
(dark	Fig (fresh/	Canang	Quince	Mango
blue/	dried)	melon	Raisin	Orange
purple)	Grapefruit	Canta-	Star fruit	Papaya
Plum	Lemon	loupe	(caram-	Plantain
Prune	Lime	Casaba	bola)	Tangerine
	Pineapple	melon	Strawberry	
		Christmas		
		melon		
		Cranberry		
		(juice)		
		Crenshaw		
		melon		
		Dewberry		
		Goose-		
		berry		
		Guava		
		Kiwi		
		Kumquat		
		Logan-		
		berry		
		Mulberry		

SUPER BENEFICIAL	BENEFICIAL	NEUTRAL: Allowed Frequently	NEUTRAL: Allowed Infrequently	AVOID
		Muskmelon		
		Nectarine		
		Peach		
		Pear		
		Persian melon		
		Persimmon		
		Prickly pear		
		Raspberry		
		Sago palm		
		Spanish melon		
		Watermelon		
		Youngberry		

Special Variants: *Non-Secretor:* BENEFICIAL: cranberry (juice), elderberry (dark blue/purple), watermelon; NEUTRAL (Allowed Frequently): banana, coconut, lime, mango, plantain, tangerine; AVOID: cantaloupe, casaba melon.

Spices/Condiments/Sweeteners

Many spices have medicinal properties. Turmeric improves liver function. Garlic improves immune health and is anti-inflammatory. Ginger aids digestive health. Many common food additives, such as guar gum and carrageenan, enhance the effects of lectins found in other foods and should be avoided.

SUPER BENEFICIAL	BENEFICIAL	NEUTRAL: Allowed Frequently	NEUTRAL: Allowed Infrequently	AVOID
Garlic	Barley malt	Agar	Brown rice	Aspartame
Ginger	Coriander	Allspice	syrup	Capers
Turmeric	seeds	Almond	Chocolate	Carrageenan
	Fenugreek	extract	Cornstarch	Chili
	Horse-	Anise	Corn syrup	powder
	radish	Apple	Dextrose	Gelatin
	Molasses	pectin	Fructose	(except
	(black-	Arrowroot	Guarana	veg-
	strap)	Basil	Honey	sourced)
	Mustard	Bay leaf	Maltodex-	Gums
	(dry)	Bergamot	trin	(acacia/
	Parsley	Caraway	Maple	Arabic/
	Soy sauce	Cardamon	syrup	guar)
	Tamari	Carob	Rice syrup	Juniper
	(wheat-	Chervil	Senna	Ketchup
	free)	Chive	Sugar	Mayonnaise
		Cilantro	(brown/	MSG
		(coriander	white)	Pepper
		leaf)		(black/
		Cinnamon		white)
		Clove		Pepper
		Cream of		(cayenne)
		tartar		Pepper (pep-
		Cumin		percorn/
		Dill		red flakes)
		Invert		Pickles/
		sugar		relish
		Licorice		Sucanat
		root*		Vinegar (all)
		Mace		Wintergreen
		Marjoram		Worcester-
		Mint (all)		shire
		Molasses		sauce

SUPER BENEFICIAL	BENEFICIAL	NEUTRAL: Allowed Frequently	NEUTRAL: Allowed Infrequently	AVOID
		Nutmeg		
		Oregano		
		Paprika		
		Rosemary		
		Saffron		
		Sage		
		Savory		
		Sea salt		
		Seaweeds		
		Stevia		
		Tamarind		
		Tarragon		
		Thyme		
		Vanilla		
		Vegetable glycerine		
		Yeast (baker's/ brewer's)		

Special Variants: *Non-Secretor:* BENEFICIAL: cilantro (coriander leaf), yeast (brewer's); NEUTRAL (Allowed Frequently): barley malt, chili powder, molasses (not blackstrap), parsley, rice syrup, soy sauce, tamari (wheat-free), turmeric, wintergreen; AVOID: agar, cornstarch, corn syrup, dextrose, invert sugar, maltodextrin, senna.

*Do not use if you have high blood pressure.

Herbal Teas

Herbal teas can provide health benefits for Blood Type A. SUPER BENEFICIAL are chamomile and holy basil, which can reduce stress; dandelion and ginger, which aid digestion; and echinacea and rosehip, which can support immune health.

SUPER BENEFICIAL	BENEFICIAL	NEUTRAL: Allowed Frequently	NEUTRAL: Allowed Infrequently	AVOID
Chamomile	Alfalfa	Chickweed	Hops	Catnip
Dandelion	Aloe	Coltsfoot	Senna	Cayenne
Echinacea	Burdock	Dong quai		Corn silk
Ginger	Fenugreek	Elderberry		Red clover
Holy basil	Gentian	Goldenseal		Rhubarb
Rosehip	Ginkgo biloba	Horehound		Yellow dock
	Ginseng	Licorice root*		
	Hawthorn	Linden		
	Milk thistle	Mulberry		
	Parsley	Mullein		
	Slippery elm	Peppermint		
	St. John's wort	Raspberry leaf		
	Stone root	Sage		
	Valerian	Sarsaparilla		
		Shepherd's purse		
		Skullcap		
		Spearmint		
		Strawberry leaf		
		Thyme		
		White birch		
		White oak bark		
		Yarrow		

Special Variants: *Non-Secretor*: AVOID: senna.

*Do not use if you have high blood pressure.

Miscellaneous Beverages

Green tea is a SUPER BENEFICIAL beverage for Blood Type A because of its antioxidant and cardiovascular properties. Red wine contains gallic acid, trans-resveratrol, quercetin, and rutin—four phenolic compounds with potent antioxidant effects.

Coffee can be consumed in moderation, as it contains enzymes also found in soy. Limit your intake if you have hot flashes. Blood Type A individuals who are not caffeine sensitive might consider having one cup of coffee daily; it contains many enzymes also found in soy, which can help the immune system function more effectively.

SUPER BENEFICIAL	BENEFICIAL	NEUTRAL: Allowed Frequently	NEUTRAL: Allowed Infrequently	AVOID
Tea (green)	Coffee (regular) Wine (red)	Coffee (decaf) Wine (white)		Beer Liquor Seltzer Soda (club) Soda (cola/ diet/misc.) Tea, black (reg/ decaf)

Special Variants: *Non-Secretor:* BENEFICIAL: wine (white); NEUTRAL (Allowed Frequently): beer, seltzer, soda (club), tea, black (reg/decaf).

Supplements

THE BLOOD TYPE A DIET offers abundant quantities of important nutrients, such as protein and iron. It is important to get as many nutrients as possible from fresh foods and use supplements only to fill in the minor deficiencies in your diet. The following supplement protocols are designed for Blood Type A women to support health during and after menopause.

Note: If you are being treated for a medical condition, consult your doctor before taking any supplements.

Blood Type A:
Basic Menopausal Support Protocol

Use this protocol for 6 weeks.

SUPPLEMENT	ACTION	DOSAGE
High-quality multiple vitamin complex (preferably blood type–specific)	Supports general health	As directed
High-quality mineral supplement (preferably blood type–specific)	Supports general health	As directed
Black cohosh (*Cimicifuga racemosa*) standardized to 2.5% triterpene glycosides	Relieves menopausal symptoms, especially hot flashes	1–2 capsules, twice daily
Squaw vine (*Mitchella repens*)	Relieves menopausal symptoms	Tincture: 10 drops in warm water, twice daily
Soy isoflavones*	Potent phytoestrogen protects against cancer; reduces menopausal symptoms	50 mg, 1 capsule daily
Pyridoxine (vitamin B$_6$)	Supports nervous system health and mental function	50 mg daily
Chamomile tea (*Matricaria chamomilla*)	Antistress and sleep aid	1–3 cups daily

*Use under supervision of a skilled practitioner.

Blood Type A:
Bone and Structural Support Protocol

Use this protocol for 6 weeks		
SUPPLEMENT	ACTION	DOSAGE
Drynaria *spp*	In traditional Chinese medicine, one of the most important herbs that can be used to heal damaged bones and ligaments; literal Chinese name means "mender of shattered bones"; appears to decrease the activity of bone-reabsorbing cells called osteoclasts	50–250 mg, once or twice daily
High-quality mineral supplement (preferably blood type–specific)	Supports general health	As directed
Calcium (from sea plants)	Maintains bone strength	1,000 mg daily
Vitamin A	Antioxidant immune support; necessary for bone health	10,000 IU, 1 capsule daily
Boron	Helps maintain healthy bones; enhances the metabolism of calcium, magnesium, copper, phosphorus, and vitamin D	1 mg, 1 capsule daily

Blood Type A:
Cardiovascular Fitness Protocol

Use this protocol for 6 weeks		
SUPPLEMENT	**ACTION**	**DOSAGE**
Pantethine (active vitamin B₅)	Lowers cholesterol	500 mg, twice daily
Ginkgo (*Ginkgo biloba*)	Increases cerebral circulation	Standardized extract: 60 mg daily
Artichoke leaf (*Cynara scolymnus*)	Enhances liver function	500 mg, twice daily
Gotu kola (*Centella asiatica*)	Improves arterial flow	100 mg, twice daily
Dandelion (*Taraxacum officinale*)	Aids metabolic balance	250 mg, twice daily

Blood Type A:
Skin Health and Vitality Protocol

Use this protocol for 4 weeks		
SUPPLEMENT	**ACTION**	**DOSAGE**
Probiotic (preferably blood type–specific)	Improves intestinal health; promotes detoxification	As directed
Vitamin A	Antioxidant; reduces oxidative damage	10,000 IU, 1 capsule daily
Pantethine (active vitamin B₅)	Balances adrenal activity; reduces the effects of stress	500 mg, 1 capsule, twice daily
Burdock root (*Artium sp*) tea	Purifies the blood; supports healthy immune function	1–3 cups daily

SUPPLEMENT	ACTION	DOSAGE
(Non-secretors) Tea tree (*Leptospermum sp*) oil lotion (5%)	Treatment of acne, eczema, and fungal infections	Apply topically, twice daily, as needed

---

GENERAL RECOMMENDATIONS USABLE BY ALL GROUPS

Topical treatment with witch hazel (*Hammamelis virginiana*) as needed

Topical treatment with Marigold juice (*Calendula officinalis*) as needed

Zinc, 15 mg: 1 capsule, twice daily

Niacinamide cream (4%): apply topically, twice daily

The Exercise Component

FOR BLOOD TYPE A, overall fitness and immune health depend on engaging in regular physical activity, with an emphasis on calming exercises such as hatha yoga and tai chi, as well as light aerobic exercise such as walking.

The following comprises the ideal exercise regimen for Blood Type A:

EXERCISE	DURATION	FREQUENCY
Hatha yoga	40–50 minutes	3–4 x week
T'ai Chi	40–50 minutes	3–4 x week
Aerobics (low impact)	40–50 minutes	2–3 x week
Treadmill	30 minutes	2–3 x week
Pilates	40–50 minutes	3–4 x week
Weight training (5–10 lb free weights)	15 minutes	2–3 x week

EXERCISE	DURATION	FREQUENCY
Cycling (recumbent bike)	30 minutes	2–3 x week
Swimming	30 minutes	2–3 x week
Brisk walking	45 minutes	2–3 x week

3 Steps to Effective Exercise

1. Warm up with stretching and flexibility moves before you start your aerobic exercise.
2. To achieve maximum cardiovascular benefits, work toward an elevated heart rate that is about 70 percent of your capacity. Once you reach the elevated rate, continue exercising to maintain that rate for twenty to thirty minutes. To calculate your maximum heart rate and performance level:
   - Subtract your age from 220.
   - Multiply the difference by .70 (or .60 if you are over age sixty). This is the high end of your performance.
   - Multiply the remainder by .50. This is the low end of your performance.
3. Finish each aerobic session with at least a five-minute cooldown of stretching and relaxation moves.

Getting Started: The First Month

IF YOU ARE NEW to the Blood Type Diet, the following guidelines will introduce you to the Blood Type A regimen over a period of one month. Follow these recommendations as closely as possible, using a notebook to record your personal experiences with the diet. In addition to factors that are measurable in laboratory tests, take the time to note changes in your energy levels, sleep patterns, digestion, and overall well-being.

I advise that you keep a daily journal of your symptoms, the times they occur, and the circumstances. This will help you better manage them. If you are experiencing perimenopause, keep a record of your cycles and the changes you notice.

Blood Type A Diet Checklist for the Menopausal Woman

Avoid or limit animal proteins. They are hard for Blood Type A to fully digest. ☐

Derive your primary protein from plant foods with seafood used occasionally. ☐

Seafood should be primarily richly oiled cold-water fish. ☐

Include modest amounts of cultured dairy foods in your diet but avoid fresh milk products. ☐

Don't overdo the grains, especially wheat-derived foods. ☐

Eat lots of BENEFICIAL fruits and vegetables, especially those high in antioxidants and fiber. ☐

Drink green tea every day for extra immune system benefits. ☐

Week 1

Blood Type Diet and Supplements

- Eliminate your most harmful AVOID foods—red meat, most dairy, and negative lectin–containing nuts, beans, and seeds.
- Include your most important BENEFICIAL foods frequently throughout the week. For example, have soy-based foods 5 times, and omega-3-rich fish 3 to 4 times, with lots of BENEFICIAL vegetables and fruits.
- Incorporate at least 1 SUPER BENEFICIAL into your daily diet. For example, have a bowl of cherries as a snack, or a spinach salad with walnuts.
- Drink 2 to 3 cups of green tea every day.

Exercise Regimen

- Plan to exercise at least 4 days this week, for 45 minutes each day.

  2 days: walking or light aerobic activity

  2 days: yoga or T'ai Chi

- If you are ill, have low energy, or are not used to exercising, start slowly and gradually increase your duration and intensity of activity. The important factor is consistency. Just do it—as much as you're able.

- Use your journal to detail the time, activity, and distance. Note the number of repetitions for each exercise.

▪ WEEK 1 SUCCESS STRATEGY ▪
Get the Most Accurate Mammogram

There is a lot of concern about whether women are getting the most accurate mammogram readings. Here are some steps you can take to improve the accuracy of your breast cancer screening test:

- Try to go to the same breast cancer screening clinic year after year.
- If you change your clinic, try to obtain the X-ray film so there will be a point of comparison.
- If you are still menstruating, wait until after your period to get a mammogram. Your breast tissue undergoes changes during your period.
- Alert the radiologist if you take hormone replacement therapy, which can make your breast tissue denser and harder to read. Some radiologists use ultrasound in combination with mammograms to get the most accurate reading.

Week 2

Blood Type Diet and Supplements

- Begin to eliminate the next level of AVOID foods—grains, vegetables, and fruits that react poorly with Type A blood.
- Eat 2 to 3 BENEFICIAL proteins every day, with special emphasis on soy. Eat omega-3-rich fish at least 3 times a week.

- Continue to Incorporate SUPER BENEFICIAL foods into your daily diet.
- Choose the NEUTRAL foods listed as "Allowed Frequently" over those listed as "Allowed Infrequently."
- Manage your mealtimes to aid proper digestion. Avoid eating on the run. Make your meals relaxing, sit-down affairs. Eat slowly and chew thoroughly to encourage digestive secretions.

Exercise Regimen

- Continue to exercise at least 4 days this week, for 45 minutes each day.

  2 days: walking or light aerobic activity

  2 days: yoga or T'ai Chi

- If your work is sedentary, get in the habit of taking a couple of "movement" breaks during the day. Walk around the block or up and down stairs.

■ WEEK 2 SUCCESS STRATEGY ■
Reduce Stress with Chi Breathing

Chi breathing is based upon the Taoist concept of Qi Gong, which represents energy as flowing according to certain routes in your body. Positive release is accessible through refining the breath. The calming, stress-relieving effects of this exercise are remarkable. It can be performed by anyone, regardless of age, fitness, or medical condition.

1. Stand comfortably, feet shoulder-width apart, knees slightly bent, arms at your side. Relax your neck and shoulder muscles and focus on your solar plexus (center of the body). It is okay to sway a bit—that's normal.
2. Start to rock back and forth gently. Inhale deeply as you rock forward onto the balls of your feet; exhale as you rock backward onto your heels.
3. As you inhale, lift your relaxed arms up and forward, keeping them relaxed and slightly bent. As you exhale, let your arms float down. Imagine that your hands are pulsing around an imaginary ball of energy.
4. Repeat, gradually refining the rhythm and developing the ability to "drop" your breath from the lungs to the solar plexus.

5. Repeat four to five times, then relax, letting your hands drop to your sides and closing your eyes. Concentrate on feeling relaxed and centered.

Week 3

Blood Type Diet and Supplements

- When you plan your meals for week 3, choose BENEFICIAL foods to replace NEUTRAL foods whenever possible. For example, choose tofu over chicken, or blueberries over an apple.
- Eliminate all remaining AVOID foods.
- Liberally incorporate SUPER BENEFICIAL foods into your daily diet.
- Drink 2 to 3 cups of green tea every day.

Exercise Regimen

- Continue to exercise at least 4 days this week, for 45 minutes each day.

  2 days: walking or light aerobic activity

  2 days: yoga or T'ai Chi

■ WEEK 3 SUCCESS STRATEGY ■
A Good Night's Sleep

Many women report having difficulty sleeping during menopause, and Type A might have a special susceptibility. High cortisol levels can disrupt your sleep cycle. You may have to work harder to stay energized. Try to establish a regular sleep schedule and adhere to it as closely as possible. When you have a normal sleep-wake rhythm, it reduces cortisol levels. During the day, schedule at least two breaks of twenty minutes each for complete relaxation. Combat sleep disturbances with regular exercise and a relaxing pre-bedtime routine. A light snack before bedtime will help raise your blood sugar levels and improve sleep. If these strategies don't work, ask your doctor about the following supplement:

Methylcobalamin (active vitamin B$_{12}$): 1 to 3 mg per day taken in the morning. This vitamin enables deep sleep and helps you wake feeling more rested. Methylcobalamin also helps folic acid lower homocysteine.

Week 4

Blood Type Diet and Supplements

- Continue at the week 3 level, focusing on BENEFICIAL and SUPER BENEFICIAL foods.

Exercise Regimen

- Continue at the week 3 level.
- Review your progress, noting in your journal improvements in strength and flexibility. Determine which exercise regimen has worked for you, including time of day, setting, and activity level.

■ WEEK 4 SUCCESS STRATEGY ■
Support Your Bones

Postmenopausal women naturally have a higher risk of bone loss, leading to osteoporosis, as a result of estrogen depletion. Type A women have an increased risk because of low levels of intestinal alkaline phosphatase. Repeated studies have shown that this enzyme positively impacts calcium metabolism. Furthermore, higher stomach acid predicts better calcium absorption. These factors present a special challenge for Type A women—especially if you are not using some form of estrogen replacement. To promote healthy bones:

1. Eat canned salmon and sardines with the bones.
2. Regularly consume low-fat yogurt, soy milk, and goat milk.
3. Include lots of broccoli and spinach in your diet.
4. Take a daily supplement of calcium citrate—300 to 600 mg.
5. Follow the Type A exercise regimen.

SIX

Blood Type

B

BLOOD TYPE B DIET OUTCOME: FEELINGS OF FULLNESS

"Several years ago, I had my uterus and ovaries removed. Shortly there-after, I began experiencing joint pain in my fingers, wrists, knees, and feet. My hands weakened to the point where I had difficulty perform-ing certain tasks, such as lifting boxes and removing items from shelves. I didn't know what to make of the problem and thought it might be re-lated to the estrogen patch I was wearing. I went to a rheumatologist be-cause my symptoms led me to believe I had arthritis. Three hundred dollars later, a series of blood tests revealed no sign of arthritis or any re-lated illness. I was happy that I didn't have it, but frustrated that I had very real pain with no diagnosis.

Then a friend sang the praises of your book, and I went out the same day to purchase it. I read all the chapters that pertain to Type Bs before beginning to make changes in my diet. I thought it would be hard, but the diet was remarkably easy to follow. For the first time in my life, I sense a true feeling of fullness, I do not eat out of nervousness, and I don't even think about food unless I am really hungry. I have had a weight problem all my life, but now I believe I will lose weight with-out any effort because I stop eating when I am full. I have lost six pounds so far. Most important, my joint pain has decreased, and this morning was the first time I got up without noticing whether my hands, knees, and feet hurt. Thank you for what seems to be a real breakthrough in health, nutrition, and weight control."

Self-reported outcomes from the Blood Type Diet Web site (www.dadamo.com).

Blood Type B: The Foods

THE BLOOD TYPE B Menopause Diet is specifically adapted to provide the maximum nutritional support to protect your health and fight the symptoms of menopause. A new category, **Super Beneficial**, highlights powerful disease-fighting foods for Blood Type B. The **Neutral** category has also been adjusted to de-emphasize foods that are less advantageous for you. Foods designated **Neutral: Allowed Infrequently** should be minimized or avoided entirely.

Your secretor status can influence your ability to fully digest and metabolize certain foods, so various adjustments in the values are made for non-secretors. If you do not know your secretor type, the odds are that you can safely use the "secretor" values, since the majority of the population (approximately 80 percent) are secretors. How-

---

Blood Type B

TOP 12 MENOPAUSE SUPER FOODS

1. lean, organic, grass-fed red meat (especially lamb and mutton)
2. richly oiled cold-water fish (halibut, sardines)
3. cultured dairy (kefir, yogurt)
4. olive oil
5. walnuts
6. flaxseeds
7. yams
8. beets
9. greens (collard, kale)
10. berries (cranberry, elderberry)
11. bananas
12. green tea

ever, I urge you to get tested, since the variations are important for non-secretors who want to maximize the effectiveness of the Blood Type Diet.

The food charts are divided into three sections. The top of the chart suggests the average portion size and quantity per week or day, according to secretor status. These recommendations do *not* apply to the category **Neutral: Allowed Infrequently**; those foods should be eaten rarely, if at all. The charts also indicate differences in frequency for some foods, based on ethnic heritage. It has been my experience that this factor has an impact upon the individual's ability to fully digest certain foods. For the purposes of blood type food choices, persons of Hispanic heritage should follow the guidelines for Caucasians, and American Native peoples should follow the guidelines for Asians.

The middle section of the chart gives the food values. The bottom section lists variants based on secretor status.

For your convenience, we have included a number of product names (Ezekiel 4:9 bread, Worcestershire sauce, etc.). However, keep in mind that commercial formulations vary among brands and regions. Even though a product may be listed as acceptable for you, always check its ingredients. Some products contain **Avoid** ingredients for your blood type. Of course, you may choose to make your own version of commercial products, such as bread and mayonnaise, using ingredients that suit your blood type. There are hundreds of delicious recipes for every blood type available on our Web site (www.dadamo.com) and in the book *Cook Right 4 Your Type: The Practical Kitchen Companion to Eat Right 4 Your Type*.

Meat/Poultry

Blood Type B is able to efficiently metabolize animal protein, but there are limitations that require careful dietary navigation. Chicken, one of the most popular food choices, disagrees with Blood Type B, because of a B-specific agglutinin, called a galectin, contained in the organ and muscle meat. This galectin can trigger inflammatory and autoimmune conditions. Turkey does not contain this lectin and can be eaten as an excellent alternative to chicken. Choose only the best quality (preferably free-range) chemical-, antibiotic-, and pesticide-free low-fat meats and poultry. Grass-fed cattle are far superior to grain-fed.

BLOOD TYPE B: MEAT/POULTRY			
Portion: 4–6 oz (men); 2–5 oz (women and children)			
	African	Caucasian	Asian
Secretor	3–6	2–6	2–5
Non-Secretor	4–7	4–7	4–7
		Times per week	

SUPER BENEFICIAL	BENEFICIAL	NEUTRAL: Allowed Frequently	NEUTRAL: Allowed Infrequently	AVOID
Goat Lamb Mutton	Rabbit Venison	Beef Buffalo Liver (calf) Ostrich Pheasant Turkey Veal		All commercially processed meats Bacon/ham/pork Chicken Cornish hen Duck Goose Grouse Guinea hen Heart (beef) Horse Partridge

SUPER BENEFICIAL	BENEFICIAL	NEUTRAL: Allowed Frequently	NEUTRAL: Allowed Infrequently	AVOID
				Quail
				Squab
				Squirrel
				Sweet-breads
				Turtle

Special Variants: *Non-Secretor:* BENEFICIAL: liver (calf); NEUTRAL (Allowed Frequently): heart (beef), horse, squab, sweetbreads.

Fish/Seafood

Richly oiled cold-water fish, such as halibut, mackerel, cod, salmon, and sardines, are especially good protein sources for Type B, since they are excellent sources of omega-3 fatty acids. Avoid shellfish, which can trigger allergic reactions. Salmon, halibut, and sardines are good sources of phosphorus (needed for energy production): ATP (adenosine triphosphate) and ADP (adenosine diphosphate).

BLOOD TYPE B: FISH/SEAFOOD			
Portion: 4–6 oz (men); 2–5 oz (women and children)			
	African	**Caucasian**	**Asian**
Secretor	4–5	3–5	3–5
Non-Secretor	4–5	4–5	4–5
	Times per week		

SUPER BENEFICIAL	BENEFICIAL	NEUTRAL: Allowed Frequently	NEUTRAL: Allowed Infrequently	AVOID
Cod	Caviar (sturgeon)	Abalone	Herring (pickled/smoked)	Anchovy
Halibut	Croaker	Bluefish	Salmon (smoked)	Barracuda
Mackerel	Flounder	Bullhead	Scallops	Bass (all)
Salmon (caught, not farm raised)	Grouper	Carp		Beluga
Sardine	Haddock	Catfish		Butterfish
	Hake	Chub		Clam
	Harvest fish	Cusk		Conch
	Mahimahi	Drum		Crab
	Monkfish	Gray sole		Crayfish
	Perch (ocean)	Halfmoon fish		Eel
	Pickerel	Herring (fresh)		Frog
	Pike	Mullet		Lobster
	Porgy	Muskel-lunge		Mussel
	Shad	Opaleye		Octopus
	Sole	Orange roughy		Oysters
	Sturgeon	Parrot fish		Pollock
		Perch (silver/white/yellow)		Shrimp
		Pompano		Snail (*Helix pomatia*/escargot)
		Red snapper		Trout (all)
		Rosefish		Yellowtail
		Sailfish		
		Scrod		
		Scup		
		Shark		
		Smelt		

SUPER BENEFICIAL	BENEFICIAL	NEUTRAL: Allowed Frequently	NEUTRAL: Allowed Infrequently	AVOID
		Squid (calamari)		
		Sucker		
		Sunfish		
		Swordfish		
		Tilapia		
		Tilefish		
		Tuna		
		Weakfish		
		Whitefish		
		Whiting		

Special Variants: *Non-Secretor:* BENEFICIAL: carp; NEUTRAL (Allowed Frequently): barracuda, butterfish, caviar (sturgeon), flounder, halibut, pike, salmon (caught, not farm-raised), sole, snail (*Helix pomatia*/escargot), yellowtail; AVOID: scallops.

Dairy/Eggs

Dairy products, especially cultured dairy products, can be eaten by almost all Blood Type B secretors, and to a lesser degree by non-secretors. Cultured dairy, such as yogurt and kefir, is particularly good for Blood Type B; these foods help build a healthy intestinal environment. Ghee (clarified butter) contains BENEFICIAL fatty acids believed to promote intestinal balance. Non-secretors should be wary of eating too much cheese, as they are more sensitive to many of the microbial strains in aged cheeses. This sensitivity is greater for those of African ancestry, but the sensitivity can also be found in Caucasian and Asian populations. Cheese consumption should also be limited for those who suffer from recurrent infections or allergies, as cheese can trigger inflammation and produce excess mucus. Eggs and some dairy products are good sources of phosphorus (needed for energy production): ATP (adenosine triphosphate) and ADP (adenosine diphosphate). Do your best to find dairy products that are both hormone-free and organic.

BLOOD TYPE B: EGGS			
Portion: 1 egg			
	African	Caucasian	Asian
Secretor	3–4	3–4	3–4
Non-Secretor	5–6	5–6	5–6
		Times per week	

BLOOD TYPE B: MILK AND YOGURT			
Portion: 4–6 oz (men); 2–5 oz (women and children)			
	African	Caucasian	Asian
Secretor	3–5	3–4	3–4
Non-Secretor	1–3	2–4	1–3
		Times per week	

BLOOD TYPE B: CHEESE			
Portion: 3 oz (men); 2 oz (women and children)			
	African	Caucasian	Asian
Secretor	3–4	3–5	3–4
Non-Secretor	1–4	1–4	1–4
		Times per week	

SUPER BENEFICIAL	BENEFICIAL	NEUTRAL: Allowed Frequently	NEUTRAL: Allowed Infrequently	AVOID
Ghee (clarified butter)	Cottage cheese	Camembert	Brie	American cheese
Kefir	Farmer cheese	Casein	Butter	Blue cheese
Yogurt	Feta	Cream cheese	Buttermilk	Egg (duck/ goose/ quail)
	Goat cheese	Edam	Cheddar	Ice cream
	Milk (cow/ goat)	Egg (chicken)	Colby	
	Mozzarella	Emmenthal	Half-and-half	
		Gouda	Jarlsberg	
		Gruyère	Monterey Jack	

SUPER BENEFICIAL	BENEFICIAL	NEUTRAL: Allowed Frequently	NEUTRAL: Allowed Infrequently	AVOID
	Paneer Ricotta	Neufchâtel Parmesan Provolone Quark Sour cream	Muenster Sherbet Swiss cheese Whey	

Special Variants: *Non-Secretor:* BENEFICIAL: whey; NEUTRAL (Allowed Frequently): cottage cheese, milk (cow); AVOID: Camembert, cheddar, Emmenthal, Jarlsberg, Monterey Jack, Muenster, Parmesan, provolone, Swiss cheese.

Oils

Blood Type B does best on monounsaturated oils and oils rich in omega series fatty acids. Olive oil fits the bill in both regards. Constituents in olive oil, such as flavonoids, squalenes, and polyphenols, act as powerful antioxidants. It should be used as the primary cooking oil. Flax (linseed) oil is high in phytoestrogen lignans, which regulate hormonal activity and reduce menopausal symptoms.

Sesame, sunflower, and corn oils should be avoided as they contain immunoreactive proteins that impair Blood Type B digestion.

BLOOD TYPE B: OILS			
Portion: 1 tblsp			
	African	Caucasian	Asian
Secretor	5–8	5–8	5–8
Non-Secretor	3–5	3–7	3–6
	Times per week		

SUPER BENEFICIAL	BENEFICIAL	NEUTRAL: Allowed Frequently	NEUTRAL: Allowed Infrequently	AVOID
Flax (linseed) Olive		Almond Black currant seed Cod liver Evening primrose Walnut	Wheat germ	Avocado Canola Castor Coconut Corn Cottonseed Peanut Safflower Sesame Soy Sunflower

Special Variants: *Non-Secretor:* BENEFICIAL: black currant seed, walnut.

Nuts/Seeds

Nuts and seeds can be an important secondary source of protein for Blood Type B. Walnuts are highly effective in inhibiting gastrointestinal toxicity; flax (linseed) contain lignans, which regulate hormonal activity and reduce menopausal symptoms.

As with other aspects of the Blood Type B Diet plan, there are some idiosyncratic elements to the choice of seeds and nuts. Several, such as sunflower and sesame, have B-agglutinating lectins and should be avoided.

BLOOD TYPE B: NUTS/SEEDS			
Portion: Whole (handful); Nut Butters (2 tblsp)			
	African	Caucasian	Asian
Secretor	4–7	4–7	4–7
Non-Secretor	5–7	5–7	5–7
	Times per week		

SUPER BENEFICIAL	BENEFICIAL	NEUTRAL: Allowed Frequently	NEUTRAL: Allowed Infrequently	AVOID
Flax (linseed) Walnut (black)		Almond Almond butter Beechnut Brazil nut Butternut Chestnut Hickory Walnut (English)	Lychee Macadamia Pecan	Cashew Filbert (hazelnut) Peanut Peanut butter Pignolia (pine nut) Pistachio Poppy seed Pumpkin seed Safflower seed Sesame butter (tahini) Sesame seed Sunflower seed

Special Variants: *Non-Secretor:* BENEFICIAL: walnut (English); NEUTRAL (Allowed Frequently): pumpkin seed.

Beans and Legumes

Blood Type B can do well on the proteins found in many beans and legumes, although this food category does contain more than a few beans with problematic lectins. Soy products should be de-emphasized, as they are rich in a class of enzymes that can interact negatively with the B antigen. Several beans, such as mung beans, contain B-agglutinating lectins and should be avoided.

BLOOD TYPE B: BEANS AND LEGUMES			
Portion: 1 cup (cooked)			
	African	Caucasian	Asian
Secretor	5–7	5–7	5–7
Non-Secretor	3–5	3–5	3–5
		Times per week	

SUPER BENEFICIAL	BENEFICIAL	NEUTRAL: Allowed Frequently	NEUTRAL: Allowed Infrequently	AVOID
	Bean (green/ snap/ string)	Cannellini bean	Soy bean	Adzuki bean
	Fava (broad) bean	Copper bean		Black bean
	Kidney bean	Jicama bean		Black-eyed pea
	Lima bean	Pea (green/ pod/ snow)		Garbanzo (chickpea)
	Navy bean	Tamarind bean		Lentil (all)
	Northern bean	White bean		Mung bean/ sprouts
				Pinto bean
				Soy cheese
				Soy milk
				Soy, miso
				Soy, tempeh
				Soy, tofu

Special Variants: *Non-Secretor:* NEUTRAL (Allowed Frequently): bean (green/snap/string), fava (broad) bean, kidney bean, lima bean, navy bean, northern bean, soy milk; AVOID: soy bean.

Grains and Starches

Grains are a leading factor in triggering inflammatory and autoimmune conditions in Blood Type B. The wheat agglutinin is particularly harmful, as is the lectin in corn. Non-secretors have an even greater sensitivity. Sprouted grains, such as Essene bread (manna), are the exception. Sprouting makes the grains less reactive to the Type B immune system.

BLOOD TYPE B: GRAINS AND STARCHES			
Portion: ½ cup dry (grains or pastas); 1 muffin; 2 slices of bread			
	African	Caucasian	Asian
Secretor	5–7	5–9	5–9
Non-Secretor	3–5	3–5	3–5
	Times per week		

SUPER BENEFICIAL	BENEFICIAL	NEUTRAL: Allowed Frequently	NEUTRAL: Allowed Infrequently	AVOID
	Essene bread (manna)	Barley	Rice flour	Amaranth
	Ezekiel 4:9 bread	Quinoa	Soy flour/ products	Buckwheat
	Millet	Spelt flour/ products	Wheat (refined/unbleached)	Cornmeal
	Oat bran		Wheat (semolina)	Couscous
	Oat flour		Wheat (white flour)	Grits
	Oatmeal			Kamut
	Rice bran			Popcorn
	Rice cake			Rice (wild)
	Rice milk			Rye
	Spelt (whole)			Rye flour
				Soba noodles (100% buckwheat)
				Sorghum
				Tapioca
				Teff

SUPER BENEFICIAL	BENEFICIAL	NEUTRAL: Allowed Frequently	NEUTRAL: Allowed Infrequently	AVOID
				Wheat (whole) Wheat bran Wheat germ

Special Variants: *Non-Secretor:* NEUTRAL (Allowed Frequently): amaranth, Ezekiel 4:9 bread, oat (all), rice (wild), sorghum, spelt (whole), tapioca; AVOID: soy flour/products, wheat (all).

Vegetables

Super Beneficial vegetables, such as maitake and shiitake mushrooms, are rich sources of antioxidants. Broccoli contains the phytochemical indole-3-carbinol, which converts strong estrogens to less carcinogenic estrogens. Beets are natural estrogen sources. Collards, kale, and spinach are rich in antioxidants.

Tomatoes contain a lectin that reacts with the saliva and digestive juices of Blood Type B secretors, although it does not appear to react with non-secretors. Corn has B-agglutinating activity and should be avoided.

An item's value also applies to its juice, unless otherwise noted.

BLOOD TYPE B: VEGETABLES			
Portion: 1 cup, prepared (cooked or raw)			
	African	Caucasian	Asian
Secretor Super/ Beneficials	Unlimited	Unlimited	Unlimited
Secretor Neutrals	2–5	2–5	2–5
Non-Secretor Super/ Beneficials	Unlimited	Unlimited	Unlimited
Non-Secretor Neutrals	2–3	2–3	2–3
	Times per day		

SUPER BENEFICIAL	BENEFICIAL	NEUTRAL: Allowed Frequently	NEUTRAL: Allowed Infrequently	AVOID
Beet	Brussels sprouts	Alfalfa sprouts	Potato	Aloe
Beet greens	Cabbage	Arugula		Artichoke
Broccoli	Cabbage (juice)*	Asparagus		Corn
Collards	Carrot	Asparagus pea		Olive (all)
Kale	Cauliflower	Bamboo shoots		Pumpkin
Spinach	Eggplant	Bok choy		Radish/ sprouts
Mushroom (maitake/ shiitake)	Mustard greens	Carrot (juice)		Rhubarb
	Parsnip	Celeriac		Tomato
	Peppers (all)	Celery		
	Potato (sweet)	Chicory		
	Yam	Cucumber		
		Daikon radish		
		Endive		
		Escarole		
		Fennel		
		Fiddlehead fern		
		Garlic		
		Horse-radish		
		Kohlrabi		
		Leek		
		Lettuce (all)		
		Mushroom (abalone/ enoki/ oyster/		

SUPER BENEFICIAL	BENEFICIAL	NEUTRAL: Allowed Frequently	NEUTRAL: Allowed Infrequently	AVOID
		Mushroom (cont'd) porto-bello/ silver dollar/ straw/ tree ear)		
		Okra		
		Onion (all)		
		Oyster plant		
		Pickle (in brine or vinegar)		
		Poi		
		Radicchio		
		Rappini (broccoli rabe)		
		Rutabaga		
		Scallion		
		Seaweeds		
		Shallot		
		Squash (all)		
		Swiss chard		
		Taro		
		Turnip		
		Water chestnut		
		Watercress		

SUPER BENEFICIAL	BENEFICIAL	NEUTRAL: Allowed Frequently	NEUTRAL: Allowed Infrequently	AVOID
		Yucca Zucchini		

Special Variants: *Non-Secretor:* BENEFICIAL: garlic, okra, onion (all); NEUTRAL (Allowed Frequently): artichoke, cabbage*, eggplant, peppers (all), pumpkin, tomato; AVOID: potato.

*To obtain the benefits of cabbage juice, it must be consumed within one minute of juicing.

Fruits and Fruit Juices

Many Super Beneficial fruits have powerful antioxidant effects, which help to reduce infection. Elderberries are particularly effective against viral infections. Watermelon improves nitric oxide synthesis and reduces edema. Plums contain phytonutrients that reduce free radical damage. Cranberries are SUPER BENEFICIAL for Blood Type B individuals, especially non-secretors, who have a higher than average risk for urinary tract infections.

An item's value also applies to its juice, unless otherwise noted.

BLOOD TYPE B: FRUITS AND FRUIT JUICES			
Portion: 1 cup			
	African	Caucasian	Asian
Secretor	2–4	3–5	3–5
Non-Secretor	2–3	2–3	2–3
	Times per day		

SUPER BENEFICIAL	BENEFICIAL	NEUTRAL: Allowed Frequently	NEUTRAL: Allowed Infrequently	AVOID
Cranberry	Banana	Apple	Apricot	Avocado
Elderberry (dark blue/ purple)	Grape	Blackberry	Asian pear	Bitter melon
	Papaya	Blueberry	Breadfruit	Coconut
	Pineapple	Boysen-berry	Cantaloupe	Persimmon
Plum		Canang melon	Currant	Pomegranate
Watermelon		Casaba melon	Date	Prickly pear
		Cherry (all)	Fig (fresh/ dried)	Star fruit (carambola)
		Christmas melon	Honeydew	
		Crenshaw melon	Plantain	
		Dewberry	Raisin	
		Goose-berry		
		Grapefruit		
		Guava		
		Kiwi		
		Kumquat		
		Lemon		
		Lime		
		Logan-berry		
		Mango		
		Mulberry		
		Muskmelon		
		Nectarine		
		Orange		
		Peach		
		Pear		

SUPER BENEFICIAL	BENEFICIAL	NEUTRAL: Allowed Frequently	NEUTRAL: Allowed Infrequently	AVOID
		Persian melon		
		Prune		
		Quince		
		Raspberry		
		Sago palm		
		Spanish melon		
		Strawberry		
		Tangerine		
		Young- berry		

Special Variants: *Non-Secretor:* BENEFICIAL: blackberry, blueberry, boysenberry, cherry, currant, fig (dried/fresh), guava, raspberry; NEUTRAL (Allowed Frequently): banana; AVOID: cantaloupe, honeydew.

Spices/Condiments/Sweeteners

Many spices are known to have medicinal properties. Turmeric improves liver function. Ginger aids digestive health, as does cayenne pepper. Licorice provides antiviral support and is important in effectively processing cortisol. Many common food additives, such as guar gum and carrageenan, enhance the effects of lectins found in other foods and should be avoided. Use caution when using prepared condiments. Often they contain wheat.

SUPER BENEFICIAL	BENEFICIAL	NEUTRAL: Allowed Frequently	NEUTRAL: Allowed Infrequently	AVOID
Ginger	Horse-radish	Anise	Agar	Allspice
Licorice root*	Molasses (black-strap)	Apple pectin	Arrowroot	Almond extract
Pepper (cayenne)	Parsley	Basil	Chocolate	Aspartame
Turmeric		Bay leaf	Fructose	Barley malt
		Bergamot	Honey	Carrageenan
		Caper	Maple syrup	Cinnamon
		Caraway	Mayon-naise	Cornstarch
		Cardamom	Molasses	Corn syrup
		Carob	Pickle (all)	Dextrose
		Chervil	Rice syrup	Gelatin (except veg-sourced)
		Chili powder	Sugar (brown/white)	Guarana
		Chive	Tamari (wheat-free)	Gums (acacia/Arabic/guar)
		Cilantro (corian-der leaf)	Vinegar (all)	Invert sugar
		Clove		Juniper
		Coriander		Ketchup
		Cream of tartar		Maltodex-trin
		Cumin		MSG
		Dill		Pepper (black/white)
		Fenugreek		Soy sauce
		Garlic		Stevia
		Lecithin		Sucanat
		Mace		Tapioca
		Marjoram		
		Mint (all)		
		Mustard (dry)		
		Nutmeg		
		Oregano		

SUPER BENEFICIAL	BENEFICIAL	NEUTRAL: Allowed Frequently	NEUTRAL: Allowed Infrequently	AVOID
		Paprika		
		Pepper (pepper-corn/red flakes)		
		Rosemary		
		Saffron		
		Sage		
		Savory		
		Sea salt		
		Seaweeds		
		Senna		
		Tamarind		
		Tarragon		
		Thyme		
		Vanilla		
		Winter-green		
		Yeast (baker's/brewer's)		

Special Variants: *Non-Secretor:* BENEFICIAL: oregano, yeast (brewer's); NEUTRAL (Allowed Frequently): stevia; AVOID: agar, fructose, pickle relish, sugar (brown/white).

*Not to be used if you have high blood pressure.

Herbal Teas

Several herbal teas are SUPER BENEFICIAL for Blood Type B. Ginger contains pungent phenolic substances with pronounced antioxidative and anti-inflammatory activities. Sage is rich in rosmarinic acid, which acts to reduce inflammatory responses by altering the concentrations of inflammatory messaging molecules. The leaves and stems of the sage plant contain antioxidant enzymes, including superoxide dismutase (SOD) and peroxidase. When combined, these three components of sage—flavonoids, phenolic acids, and oxygen-handling enzymes—give it a unique capacity for stabilizing oxygen-related metabolism and preventing oxygen-based damage to the cells. Licorice root tea provides antiviral support for Blood Type B. Ginseng and dandelion can help reduce stress.

SUPER BENEFICIAL	BENEFICIAL	NEUTRAL: Allowed Frequently	NEUTRAL: Allowed Infrequently	AVOID
Dandelion	Parsley	Alfalfa		Aloe
Ginger	Peppermint	Burdock		Coltsfoot
Ginseng	Raspberry	Catnip		Corn silk
Licorice root*	leaf	Chamomile		Fenugreek
Sage	Rosehip	Chickweed		Gentian
		Dong quai		Hops
		Echinacea		Linden
		Elder		Mullein
		Goldenseal		Red clover
		Hawthorn		Rhubarb
		Horehound		Shepherd's purse
		Mulberry		Skullcap
		Rosemary		
		Sarsaparilla		
		Senna		
		Slippery elm		
		Spearmint		
		St. John's wort		
		Strawberry leaf		

SUPER BENEFICIAL	BENEFICIAL	NEUTRAL: Allowed Frequently	NEUTRAL: Allowed Infrequently	AVOID
		Thyme		
		Valerian		
		Vervain		
		White birch		
		White oak bark		
		Yarrow		
		Yellow dock		

Special Variants: None.

*Not to be used if you have high blood pressure.

Miscellaneous Beverages

Green tea should be part of every Blood Type B's health plan. It contains polyphenols, which enhance gastrointestinal health. Alcohol can exacerbate autoimmune inflammatory conditions. Avoid or limit alcohol to an occasional glass of red wine. If you are a heavy coffee drinker, try to reduce your intake or slowly eliminate it altogether, especially if you are having hot flashes.

SUPER BENEFICIAL	BENEFICIAL	NEUTRAL: Allowed Frequently	NEUTRAL: Allowed Infrequently	AVOID
Tea (green)		Wine (red/ white)	Beer	Liquor
			Coffee (reg/ decaf)	Seltzer
				Soda (club)
				Soda (cola/ diet/misc.)

SUPER BENEFICIAL	BENEFICIAL	NEUTRAL: Allowed Frequently	NEUTRAL: Allowed Infrequently	AVOID
			Tea, black (reg/ decaf)	

Special Variants: *Non-Secretor:* BENEFICIAL: wine (red/white); NEUTRAL (Allowed Frequently): liquor, seltzer, soda (club); AVOID: coffee (reg/decaf), tea, black (reg/ decaf).

Supplements

THE BLOOD TYPE B DIET offers abundant quantities of important nutrients, such as protein and iron. It is important to get as many nutrients as possible from fresh foods and use supplements only to fill in the minor deficiencies in your diet. The following supplement protocols are designed for Blood Type B women to support health during and after menopause.

Note: If you are being treated for a medical condition, consult your doctor before taking any supplements.

Blood Type B: Basic Menopausal Support Protocol

Use this protocol for 6 weeks		
SUPPLEMENT	**ACTION**	**DOSAGE**
High-quality multiple vitamin complex (preferably blood type–specific)	Supports general health	As directed
Motherwort (*Leonurus cardiaca*)	Relieves menopausal symptoms	Tincture: 10–15 drops daily
Methylcobalamin (active vitamin B_{12})	Supports nervous system health	400 mcg, 1 capsule before bed

SUPPLEMENT	ACTION	DOSAGE
Dong quai (*Angelica sinensis*)	Relieves menopausal symptoms	250 mg, 1–2 capsules daily

Blood Type B: Bone and Structural Support Protocol

Use this protocol for 6 weeks		
SUPPLEMENT	ACTION	DOSAGE
High-quality mineral supplement (preferably blood type–specific)	Supports general health	As directed
Magnesium	Necessary for bone health and calcium absorption	350 mg, 2 capsules, twice daily
Vitamin A	Antioxidant immune support; necessary for bone health	10,000 IU, 1 capsule daily
Boron	Helps maintain healthy bones; enhances the metabolism of calcium, magnesium, copper, phosphorus, and vitamin D	1 mg, 1 capsule daily

Blood Type B: Cardiovascular Fitnesss Protocol

Use this protocol for 6 weeks		
SUPPLEMENT	ACTION	DOSAGE
OPCs (oligomeric proanthocyanidins)	Have antioxidant effects	100 mg daily
Alpha-lipoic acid	Enhances insulin metabolism	50 mg daily
Curcumin (Turmeric: *Curcuma longa*)	Improves cardiac health; protects the liver	300–500 mg, 1–2 capsules daily

SUPPLEMENT	ACTION	DOSAGE
Fenugreek (*Trigonella foenum-graecum*)	Improves insulin production; reduces triglycerides	500 mg, twice daily
Larch arabinogalactan (*Larix officinalis*)	Promotes digestive and intestinal health	1 tablespoon, twice daily, in juice or water

Blood Type B: Skin Health and Vitality Protocol

Use this protocol for 4 weeks

SUPPLEMENT	ACTION	DOSAGE
OPCs (oligomeric proanthocyanidins)	Have antioxidant effects	100 mg daily
Sarsaparilla (*Smilax officinalis*)	General skin tonic	250 mg, 1–2 capsules daily
Pantothenic acid (vitamin B$_5$)	Balances adrenal activity and reduces the effects of stress; reduces allergic reactions	500 mg, twice daily
(Non-secretors) Tea tree (*Leptospermum sp*) oil lotion (5%)	Treatment of acne, eczema, and fungal infections	Apply topically, twice daily, as needed

---

GENERAL RECOMMENDATIONS USABLE BY ALL GROUPS

Topical treatment with witch hazel (*Hamamelis virginiana*) as needed

Topical treatment with marigold juice (*Calendula officinalis*) as needed

Zinc, 15 mg: 1 capsule, twice daily

Niacinamide cream (4%): apply topically, twice daily

The Exercise Component

FOR BLOOD TYPE B, stress regulation and overall fitness are achieved with a balance of moderate aerobic activity and mentally soothing, stress-reducing exercises. Below is a list of exercises that are recommended for Blood Type B.

EXERCISE	DURATION	FREQUENCY
Tennis	45–60 minutes	2–3 x week
Martial arts	30–60 minutes	2–3 x week
Cycling	45–60 minutes	2–3 x week
Hiking	30–60 minutes	2–3 x week
Golf (no cart!)	60–90 minutes	2–3 x week
Running or brisk walking	40–50 minutes	2–3 x week
Pilates	40–50 minutes	2–3 x week
Swimming	45 minutes	2–3 x week
Yoga	40–50 minutes	1–2 x week
T'ai Chi	40–50 minutes	1–2 x week

3 Steps to Effective Exercise

1. Warm up with stretching and flexibility moves before you start your aerobic exercise.
2. To achieve maximum cardiovascular benefits, work toward an elevated heart rate that is about 70 percent of your capacity. Once you reach the elevated rate, continue exercising to maintain that rate for twenty to thirty minutes. To calculate your maximum heart rate and performance level:
   • Subtract your age from 220.
   • Multiply the difference by .70 (or .60 if you are over age sixty). This is the high end of your performance.
   • Multiply the remainder by .50. This is the low end of your performance.
3. Finish each aerobic session with at least a five-minute cooldown of stretching and relaxation moves.

Getting Started: The First Month

IF YOU ARE NEW to the Blood Type Diet, the following guidelines will introduce you to the Blood Type B regimen over a period of one month. Follow these recommendations as closely as possible, using a notebook to record your personal experiences with the diet. In addition to factors that are measurable in laboratory tests, take the time to note changes in your energy levels, sleep patterns, digestion, and overall well-being.

I advise that you keep a daily journal of your symptoms, the times they occur, and the circumstances. This will help you better manage them. If you are experiencing perimenopause, keep a record of your cycles and the changes you notice.

Blood Type B Diet Checklist for the Menopausal Woman

Eat small to moderate portions of high-quality, lean, organic meat (especially goat, lamb, and mutton) several times a week for strength, energy, and digestive health. ☐

Avoid chicken. ☐

Include regular portions of richly oiled cold-water fish. ☐

Regularly eat cultured dairy foods, such as yogurt and kefir, which are BENEFICIAL for digestive health. ☐

Eliminate wheat and corn from your diet. ☐

Eat lots of BENEFICIAL fruits and vegetables. ☐

If you need a daily dose of caffeine, replace coffee with green tea. ☐

Avoid foods that are Type B red flags, especially chicken, corn, buckwheat, peanuts, soy beans, lentils, potatoes, and tomatoes. ☐

Week 1

Blood Type Diet and Supplements

- Eliminate your most harmful AVOID foods—chicken, corn, and wheat.

- Include your most important BENEFICIAL foods on a regular schedule throughout the week. For example, have lean red meat 5 times, and omega-3-rich fish 3 to 4 times, with lots of BENEFICIAL vegetables and fruit.

- Incorporate at least 1 SUPER BENEFICIAL into your daily diet. For example, have a handful of walnuts as a snack, or eat yogurt mixed with berries for lunch.

- If you're a coffee drinker, begin to wean yourself by cutting your daily consumption in half, substituting green tea.

Exercise Regimen

- Plan to exercise at least 4 days this week, for 45 minutes each day.

  2–3 days: aerobic activity

  1–2 days: yoga or T'ai Chi

- If you have an infection or are in ill health, start slowly and gradually increase your duration and intensity of activity. The important factor is consistency. Just do it—as much as you're able.

- Use your journal to detail the time, activity, and distance. Note the number of repetitions for each exercise.

■ **WEEK 1 SUCCESS STRATEGY** ■
Soothing Soak

This neutral bath calms the nervous system. Neutral means body temperature, not hot. Mix the following herbs and tie them into a cotton scarf.

1 ounce rose
1 ounce lavender

Place the scarf over the tub nozzle. Run hot water through the herbs until the tub is half full, then add cold water to bring it to the right temperature. As the water cools while you're soaking, add more warm water.

(continued)

An alternative method is to mix a few drops of rose and lavender essential oils with a teaspoon of olive oil and pour it into the tub once the water has reached the right temperature.

Week 2

Blood Type Diet and Supplements

- Begin to eliminate the next level of AVOID foods—seeds, beans, and legumes that have negative lectin activity.
- Eat at least 2 to 3 BENEFICIAL animal proteins every day from the meat, seafood, and dairy lists.
- Initially, it is best to avoid foods on the list NEUTRAL: Allowed Infrequently.
- Continue to incorporate SUPER BENEFICIAL foods into your daily diet.
- If you're a coffee drinker, continue to cut your coffee intake, replacing it with green tea.

Exercise Regimen

- Continue to exercise at least 4 days this week, for 45 minutes each day.

  2–3 days: aerobic activity

  1–2 days: yoga or T'ai Chi
- If your work is sedentary, get in the habit of taking a couple of "movement" breaks during the day. Walk around the block or up and down stairs.

▪ WEEK 2 SUCCESS STRATEGY ▪
Do Your Kegels

If you have problems with urinary leakage, kegel exercises can help strengthen the muscles around your urethra. Here's how to do them:

Contract the muscles in your vagina, urethra, and anus—as if you were trying to hold back urine. Hold for five to seven seconds, then release. Repeat ten to twenty times a day.

Week 3

Blood Type Diet and Supplements

- When you plan your meals for week 3, choose BENEFICIAL foods to replace NEUTRAL foods whenever possible. For example, choose lamb over beef, or blueberries over an apple.
- Eliminate all remaining AVOID foods.
- Liberally incorporate SUPER BENEFICIAL foods into your daily diet.

Exercise Regimen

- Continue to exercise at least 4 days this week, for 45 minutes each day.

  2–3 days: aerobic activity

  1–2 days: yoga or T'ai Chi

■ WEEK 3 SUCCESS STRATEGY ■
Visualize Your Way to a Better Immune System

Take advantage of Blood Type B's natural ability to relieve stress through meditation or guided imagery. I've never medicated Type B individuals who have high blood pressure without first teaching them some simple visualization techniques and sending them home to try them out for a few weeks. Those that did almost never required medication. Here is a very simple visualization exercise to help control high blood pressure. Do this visualization two to four times daily for five to eight minutes.

Find a quiet place and make yourself comfortable and relaxed. Close your eyes and let your arms and hands lie limply on your sides or in your lap. Take a few deep breaths, inhaling through your nose and exhaling through your mouth, while imagining the red blood cells of your circulatory system coursing through your arteries and veins. See them slipping and sliding along the walls, which periodically open up like Venetian blinds to allow cells to move from the inside of the arteries out and from the outside in. Imagine the walls of your arteries relaxing and bending. Now expand the image and visualize your entire body. See the blood circulating from your heart to the arteries, to the capillaries, to the veins, then back to the lungs and heart.

Week 4

Blood Type Diet and Supplements

- Continue at the week 3 level, focusing on BENEFICIAL and SUPER BENEFICIAL foods.
- Evaluate the first 4 weeks and make adjustments.

Exercise Regimen

- Continue at the week 3 level.
- Review your progress, noting in your journal improvements in strength and flexibility. Determine which exercise regimen has worked for you, including time of day, setting, and activity level.

■ **WEEK 4 SUCCESS STRATEGY** ■
Dry Skin Brushing

Dry skin brushing is a method of daily hygiene that has many benefits and has been around for a long time. The skin is a major organ of the body that functions as protection and as a means of elimination. What daily skin brushing will do:

- Removes dried, dead cells that block the pores of the skin, allowing the skin to breathe easier and increasing its ability to protect and eliminate the waste products of metabolism.
- Increases circulation of the blood and lymph vessels that lie close to the surface just under the skin. The blood, fluid, and its contents are returned to the heart for redistribution and/or elimination.
- Increases the nutrients to the skin. By clearing out stagnant materials, there is an increased oxygen/carbon dioxide exchange, and other nutrients, vitamins, minerals, enzymes, etc., are also brought to the area.
- Removes waste products of cellular metabolism through the blood vessels and sweating.
- Decreases the workload on the rest of the body in regard to circulation and elimination.
- Warms the skin.

PROCEDURE

Skin brushing should be done with a natural- or nylon-bristle body brush before the bath or shower but can replace the bath if no water is available. It is suggested the brushing be done toward the heart; start with the lower limbs, arms, back, then the front of the body, using a moderate pressure with short strokes upward and inward. If you have a soft complexion brush, the face can be done as well, using more circular motions. Strokes should bring a slight pink color or tingling sensation to the skin—never bruising, scraping, bleeding, or pain. One time through for each body area is sufficient.

AVOID SKIN BRUSHING IF

- You have delicate skin.
- You have easily damaged skin.
- You have an open wound.
- You have known malignancies of the skin or lymph system.

SEVEN

Blood Type

AB

BLOOD TYPE AB DIET OUTCOME: MIRACLES HAPPEN

"I have had miraculous results with the Type AB diet. I have more energy, feel good, and most of all, no food cravings. And coming from where I come from with food and eating, this is truly remarkable. I have been a compulsive eater for over thirty years with no long-term diet success. I am slowly getting off Premarin and am choosing to use 'natural' estrogen therapy. This is the *first* thing that has ever worked for me."

Self-reported outcomes from the Blood Type Diet Web site (www.dadamo.com).

Blood Type AB: The Foods

THE BLOOD TYPE AB Menopause Diet is specifically adapted to provide the maximum nutritional support to protect your health and fight the symptoms of menopause. A new category, **Super Beneficial**, highlights powerful disease-fighting foods for Blood Type AB. The **Neutral** category has also been adjusted to de-emphasize foods that are less advantageous for you. Foods designated **Neutral: Allowed Infrequently** should be minimized or avoided entirely.

Your secretor status can influence your ability to fully digest and metabolize certain foods, so various adjustments in the values are made for non-secretors. If you do not know your secretor type, the odds are that you can safely use the "secretor" values, since the majority of the population (approximately 80 percent) are secretors. However, I urge you to get tested, since the variations are important for non-secretors who want to maximize the effectiveness of the Blood Type Diet.

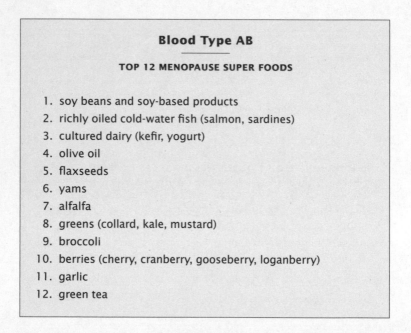

Blood Type AB

TOP 12 MENOPAUSE SUPER FOODS

1. soy beans and soy-based products
2. richly oiled cold-water fish (salmon, sardines)
3. cultured dairy (kefir, yogurt)
4. olive oil
5. flaxseeds
6. yams
7. alfalfa
8. greens (collard, kale, mustard)
9. broccoli
10. berries (cherry, cranberry, gooseberry, loganberry)
11. garlic
12. green tea

The food charts are divided into three sections. The top of the chart suggests the average portion size and quantity per week or day, according to secretor status. These recommendations do *not* apply to the category **Neutral: Allowed Infrequently**; those foods should be eaten rarely, if at all. The charts also indicate differences in frequency for some foods, based on ethnic heritage. It has been my experience that this factor has an impact upon the individual's ability to fully digest certain foods. For the purposes of blood type food choices, persons of Hispanic heritage should follow the guidelines for Caucasians, and American Native peoples should follow the guidelines for Asians.

The middle section of the chart gives the food values. The bottom section lists variants based on secretor status.

For your convenience, we have included a number of product names (Ezekiel 4:9 bread, Worcestershire sauce, etc.). However, keep in mind that commercial formulations vary among brands and regions. Even though a product may be listed as acceptable for you, always check its ingredients. Some products contain **Avoid** ingredients for your blood type. Of course, you may choose to make your own version of commercial products, such as bread and mayonnaise, using ingredients that suit your blood type. There are hundreds of delicious recipes for every blood type available on our Web site (www.dadamo.com) and in the book *Cook Right 4 Your Type: The Practical Kitchen Companion to Eat Right 4 Your Type.*

Meat/Poultry

Blood Type AB is somewhat better adapted to animal-based proteins than Blood Type A, mainly because of the B gene's effects on the production of enzymes involved in fat transport and digestion. However, Type AB should limit meat and avoid chicken, which contains a B-immunoreactive lectin. Choose only the best quality (preferably free-range) chemical-, antibiotic-, and pesticide-free low-fat meats and poultry.

BLOOD TYPE AB: MEATS/POULTRY			
Portion: 4–6 oz (men); 2–5 oz (women and children)			
	African	Caucasian	Asian
Secretor	2–5	1–5	1–5
Non-Secretor	3–5	2–5	2–5
	Times per week		

SUPER BENEFICIAL	BENEFICIAL	NEUTRAL: Allowed Frequently	NEUTRAL: Allowed Infrequently	AVOID
	Lamb Mutton Rabbit Turkey	Goat Ostrich Pheasant	Liver (calf)	All commercially processed meats Bacon/ham/pork Beef Buffalo Chicken Cornish hen Duck Goose Grouse Guinea hen Heart (beef) Partridge Quail Squab Squirrel Sweetbreads Turtle Veal Venison

Special Variants: *Non-Secretor:* NEUTRAL (Allowed Frequently): quail, venison.

Fish/Seafood

Fish and seafood provide an excellent means of optimizing NK cell activity. Richly oiled cold-water fish, such as mackerel, salmon, and sardines, are good sources of omega-3 fatty acids. They are also good food sources of phosphorus and adenosine, used to make cellular energy. In general, many of the seafoods Blood Type AB must avoid have lectins with either A or B specificity, or polyamines commonly found in the foods. Avoid consuming flash-frozen fish, which has a high polyamine content.

BLOOD TYPE AB: FISH/SEAFOOD			
Portion: 4–6 oz (men); 2–5 oz (women and children)			
	African	Caucasian	Asian
Secretor	4–6	3–5	3–5
Non-Secretor	4–7	4–6	4–6
	Times per week		

SUPER BENEFICIAL	BENEFICIAL	NEUTRAL: Allowed Frequently	NEUTRAL: Allowed Infrequently	AVOID
Mackerel	Cod	Abalone	Caviar (sturgeon)	Anchovy
Salmon (caught, not farm raised)	Grouper	Bluefish	Mussel	Barracuda
	Mahimahi	Bullhead	Scallops	Bass (all)
	Monkfish	Butterfish	Squid (calamari)	Beluga
Sardine	Pickerel	Carp	Whitefish	Clam
	Pike	Catfish		Conch
	Porgy	Chub		Crab
	Red snapper	Croaker		Eel
	Sailfish	Cusk		Flounder
	Shad	Drum		Frog
	Snail (*Helix pomatia*/ escargot)	Halfmoon fish		Gray sole
		Harvest fish		Haddock
				Hake
				Halibut

SUPER BENEFICIAL	BENEFICIAL	NEUTRAL: Allowed Frequently	NEUTRAL: Allowed Infrequently	AVOID
	Sturgeon Tuna	Herring (fresh) Mullet Muskel- lunge Opaleye Orange roughy Parrot fish Perch (all) Pollock Pompano Rosefish Scrod Scup Shark Smelt Sucker Sunfish Swordfish Tilapia Tilefish Tuna Weakfish		Herring (pickled/ smoked) Lobster Octopus Oysters Salmon (smoked) Salmon roe Shrimp Sole Trout (all) Whiting Yellowtail

Special Variants: *Non-Secretor:* BENEFICIAL: herring (fresh); NEUTRAL (Allowed Frequently): trout (all).

Dairy/Eggs

Dairy products can be used with discretion by many Blood Type AB individuals, especially secretors. Cultured dairy foods, such as yogurt and kefir, are particularly BENEFICIAL. Ghee (clarified butter) is an antioxidant rich in omega-3 oils and short-chain fatty acids. Eggs, which, like fish, are a good source of docosohexaenoic acid, can complement the protein profile for your blood type. Do your best to find eggs and dairy products that are both hormone-free and organic.

BLOOD TYPE AB: EGGS			
Portion: 1 egg			
	African	Caucasian	Asian
Secretor	2–5	3–4	3–4
Non-Secretor	3–6	3–6	3–6
	Times per week		

BLOOD TYPE AB: MILK AND YOGURT			
Portion: 4–6 oz (men); 2–5 oz (women and children)			
	African	Caucasian	Asian
Secretor	2–6	3–6	1–6
Non-Secretor	0–3	0–4	0–3
	Times per week		

BLOOD TYPE AB: CHEESE			
Portion: 3 oz (men); 2 oz (women and children)			
	African	Caucasian	Asian
Secretor	2–3	3–4	3–4
Non-Secretor	0	0–1	0
	Times per week		

SUPER BENEFICIAL	BENEFICIAL	NEUTRAL: Allowed Frequently	NEUTRAL: Allowed Infrequently	AVOID
Kefir Yogurt	Cottage cheese Egg (chicken)	Casein Cream cheese Edam	Cheddar Colby Emmenthal Milk (cow)	American cheese Blue cheese Brie Butter

SUPER BENEFICIAL	BENEFICIAL	NEUTRAL: Allowed Frequently	NEUTRAL: Allowed Infrequently	AVOID
	Farmer cheese	Egg (goose/ quail)	Monterey Jack	Buttermilk
	Feta	Ghee (clarified butter)	Sherbet	Camembert
	Goat cheese		Swiss cheese	Egg (duck)
	Milk (goat)	Gouda		Half-and-half
	Mozzarella	Gruyère		Ice cream
	Ricotta	Jarlsberg		Parmesan
	Sour cream	Muenster		Provolone
		Neufchâtel		
		Paneer		
		Quark		
		String cheese		
		Whey		

Special Variants: *Non-Secretor:* BENEFICIAL: ghee (clarified butter); NEUTRAL (Allowed Frequently): goat cheese, yogurt; AVOID: Emmenthal, Swiss cheese.

Oils

Olive oil, a monounsaturated fat, is SUPER BENEFICIAL for Blood Type AB. Constituents in olive oil, such as flavonoids, squalenes, and polyphenols, act as powerful antioxidants. It should be used as a primary cooking oil. Flax (lineseed) oil is high in phytoestrogen lignans, which regulate hormonal activity and reduce menopausal symptoms.

Corn, sesame, and safflower oils can contain immunoreactive proteins that impair Blood Type AB digestion. These oils can interfere with proper immune function.

BLOOD TYPE AB: OILS			
Portion: 1 tblsp			
	African	Caucasian	Asian
Secretor	4–7	5–8	5–7
Non-Secretor	3–6	3–6	3–4
		Times per week	

SUPER BENEFICIAL	BENEFICIAL	NEUTRAL: Allowed Frequently	NEUTRAL: Allowed Infrequently	AVOID
Flax (linseed) Olive	Walnut	Almond Black currant seed Borage seed Canola Castor Cod liver Evening primrose Peanut Soy	Wheat germ	Avocado Coconut Corn Cottonseed Safflower Sesame Sunflower

Special Variants: None.

Nuts/Seeds

Nuts and seeds can be an important secondary source of protein for Blood Type AB. Laboratory research has identified at least five natural phytochemicals in nuts that regulate the immune system and act as antioxidants. SUPER BENEFICIAL for Blood Type AB are flax (linseed) and walnuts, which are high in omega-3 fatty acids. Flax (linseed) are high in phytoestrogen lignans, which regulate hormonal activity and reduce menopausal symptoms.

BLOOD TYPE AB: NUTS/SEEDS			
Portion: Whole (handful); Nut Butters (2 tblsp)			
	African	Caucasian	Asian
Secretor	5–10	5–10	5–9
Non-Secretor	4–8	4–9	5–9
		Times per week	

SUPER BENEFICIAL	BENEFICIAL	NEUTRAL: Allowed Frequently	NEUTRAL: Allowed Infrequently	AVOID
Flax (linseed)	Chestnut	Almond	Brazil nut	Filbert (hazelnut)
Walnut (black/ English)	Peanut	Almond butter	Cashew	Poppy seed
	Peanut butter	Almond cheese	Cashew butter	Pumpkin seed
		Almond milk	Macadamia	Sesame butter (tahini)
		Beechnut	Pecan	Sesame seed
		Butternut	Pecan butter	Sunflower butter
		Hickory	Pistachio	Sunflower seed
		Lychee	Safflower seed	
		Pignolia (pine nut)		

Special Variants: *Non-Secretor:* NEUTRAL (Allowed Frequently): peanut, peanut butter; AVOID: Brazil nut, cashew, cashew butter, pistachio.

Beans and Legumes

Blood Type AB does well on proteins found in many beans and legumes, although this food category contains more than a few beans with problematic A- or B-specific lectins. In general, soy beans and their related products are SUPER BENEFICIAL. In particular, soy beans are beneficial for menopausal women. They contain isoflavones that help minimize symptoms, build bone, and protect against cancer. Soy isoflavones also inhibit the enzyme aromatase (which converts steroids to estrogens) and so help build lean muscle mass.

BLOOD TYPE AB: BEANS AND LEGUMES			
Portion: 1 cup (cooked)			
	African	**Caucasian**	**Asian**
Secretor	3–6	3–6	4–6
Non-Secretor	2–5	2–5	3–6
	Times per week		

SUPER BENEFICIAL	BENEFICIAL	NEUTRAL: Allowed Frequently	NEUTRAL: Allowed Infrequently	AVOID
Soy bean Soy cheese Soy milk Soy, miso Soy, tempeh Soy, tofu	Lentil (green) Navy bean Pinto bean	Bean (green/ snap/ string) Cannellini bean Copper bean Lentil (domestic/ red) Northern bean Pea (green/ pod/ snow) Tamarind bean White bean	Jicama bean	Adzuki bean Black bean Black-eyed pea Fava (broad) bean Garbanzo (chickpea) Kidney bean Lima bean Mung bean/ sprouts

Special Variants: *Non-Secretor:* NEUTRAL (Allowed Frequently): fava (broad) bean, navy bean, soy bean, soy (miso), soy (tempeh), soy (tofu), AVOID; jicama bean, soy cheese, soy milk.

Grains and Starches

Blood Type AB benefits from a moderate consumption of the proper grains for its blood type. Essene (manna) bread is SUPER BENEFICIAL. It is a 100 percent sprouted bread, from which the lectin-containing seed coat has been removed. Blood Type AB individuals—especially non-secretors—should use Essene instead of other wheat breads. Blood Type AB is also sensitive to the lectin in corn and should avoid all corn flour products.

BLOOD TYPE AB: GRAINS AND STARCHES			
Portion: ½ cup dry (grains or pastas); 1 muffin; 2 slices of bread			
	African	Caucasian	Asian
Secretor	6–8	6–9	6–10
Non-Secretor	4–6	5–7	6–8
		Times per week	

SUPER BENEFICIAL	BENEFICIAL	NEUTRAL: Allowed Frequently	NEUTRAL: Allowed Infrequently	AVOID
Essene bread (manna)	Amaranth	Barley	Wheat (semolina)	Buckwheat
Soy flour/ products	Ezekiel 4:9 bread	Couscous	Wheat (whole)	Cornmeal
	Millet	Quinoa	Wheat bran	Grits
	Oat bran	Spelt flour/ products	Wheat germ	Kamut
	Oat flour			Popcorn
	Oatmeal			Soba noodles (100% buckwheat)
	Rice (whole)			Sorghum
	Rice (wild)			Tapioca
	Rice bran			Teff
	Rice cake			
	Rye (whole)			

SUPER BENEFICIAL	BENEFICIAL	NEUTRAL: Allowed Frequently	NEUTRAL: Allowed Infrequently	AVOID
	Rye flour/ products Spelt (whole)			Wheat (refined/unbleached) Wheat (white flour)

Special Variants: *Non-Secretor:* NEUTRAL (Allowed Frequently): Ezekiel 4:9 bread, spelt (whole); AVOID: soy flour/products, wheat (semolina), wheat (whole), wheat germ.

Vegetables

SUPER BENEFICIAL vegetables, such as maitake and shiitake mushrooms, are rich sources of antioxidants. Broccoli contains the phytochemical indole-3-carbinol, which converts strong estrogens to less carcinogenic estrogens. Beets are natural estrogen sources. Collards, kale, beet greens, and spinach are rich in antioxidants. Alfalfa sprouts are a good source of phytoestrogens.

An item's value also applies to its juice, unless otherwise noted.

BLOOD TYPE AB: VEGETABLES			
Portion: 1 cup, prepared (cooked or raw)			
	African	Caucasian	Asian
Secretor Super/ Beneficials	Unlimited	Unlimited	Unlimited
Secretor Neutrals	2–5	2–5	2–5
Non-Secretor Super/Beneficials	Unlimited	Unlimited	Unlimited
Non-Secretor Neutrals	2–3	2–3	2–3
	Times per day		

SUPER BENEFICIAL	BENEFICIAL	NEUTRAL: Allowed Frequently	NEUTRAL: Allowed Infrequently	AVOID
Alfalfa sprouts	Cabbage (juice)*	Arugula	Carrot	Aloe
Beet	Carrot (juice)	Asparagus	Daikon radish	Artichoke
Beet greens	Cauliflower	Asparagus pea	Olive (Greek/ green/ Spanish)	Corn
Broccoli	Celery	Bamboo shoot		Mushroom (abalone/ shiitake)
Mushroom (maitake/ silver dollar)	Collards	Bok choy	Poi	Olive (black)
	Cucumber	Brussels sprouts	Potato	Peppers (all)
	Eggplant	Cabbage	Pumpkin	Pickle (all)
	Garlic	Celeriac	Taro	Radish/ sprouts
	Kale	Chicory		Rhubarb
	Mustard greens	Cucumber (juice)		
	Onion (all)	Endive		
	Parsnip	Escarole		
	Potato (sweet)	Fennel		
	Spinach	Fiddlehead fern		
	Yam	Horse- radish		
		Kohlrabi		
		Leek		
		Lettuce (all)		
		Mushroom (enoki/ oyster/ porto- bello/ silver dollar/ straw/ tree ear)		

SUPER BENEFICIAL	BENEFICIAL	NEUTRAL: Allowed Frequently	NEUTRAL: Allowed Infrequently	AVOID
		Okra		
		Oyster plant		
		Radicchio		
		Rappini (broccoli rabe)		
		Rutabaga		
		Scallion		
		Seaweeds		
		Shallot		
		Squash (all)		
		Swiss chard		
		Tomato		
		Turnip		
		Water chestnut		
		Watercress		
		Yucca		
		Zucchini		

Special Variants: *Non-Secretor:* BENEFICIAL: tomato; NEUTRAL (Allowed Frequently): beet; AVOID: poi, taro.

*To obtain the benefits of cabbage juice, it must be consumed within one minute of juicing.

Fruits and Fruit Juices

SUPER BENEFICIAL fruits for Blood Type AB include cherries, which contain pigments that inhibit intestinal toxins, and cranberries, which can help fight urinary tract infections. Many fruits, such as pineapple, are rich in enzymes that can help reduce inflammation and encourage proper water balance. Grapes and grape juice are powerful antioxidants.

An item's value also applies to its juice, unless otherwise noted.

BLOOD TYPE AB: FRUITS AND FRUIT JUICES			
Portion: 1 cup			
	African	**Caucasian**	**Asian**
Secretor	3–4	3–6	3–5
Non-Secretor	1–3	2–3	3–4
		Times per day	

SUPER BENEFICIAL	BENEFICIAL	NEUTRAL: Allowed Frequently	NEUTRAL: Allowed Infrequently	AVOID
Cherry	Fig (fresh/	Apple	Apricot	Avocado
Cranberry	dried)	Blackberry	Asian pear	Banana
Grape (all)	Gooseberry	Blueberry	Breadfruit	Bitter melon
Pineapple	Grapefruit	Boysen-	Canang	Coconut
	Kiwi	berry	melon	Dewberry
	Lemon	Elderberry	Cantaloupe	Guava
	Loganberry	(dark	Casaba	Mango
	Plum	blue/	melon	Orange
	Water-	purple)	Christmas	Persimmon
	melon	Grapefruit	melon	Pomegranate
		(juice)	Crenshaw	Prickly pear
		Kumquat	melon	Quince
		Lime	Currant	Sago palm
		Mulberry	Date	Star fruit
		Muskmelon	Honeydew	(carambola)
		Nectarine	Prune	
		Papaya	Raisin	
		Peach	Tangerine	

SUPER BENEFICIAL	BENEFICIAL	NEUTRAL: Allowed Frequently	NEUTRAL: Allowed Infrequently	AVOID
		Pear		
		Persian melon		
		Pineapple (juice)		
		Plantain		
		Raspberry		
		Spanish melon		
		Strawberry		
		Young-berry		

Special Variants: *Non-Secretor:* BENEFICIAL: blackberry, blueberry, elderberry, lime; NEUTRAL (Allowed Frequently): banana; AVOID: cantaloupe, honeydew, prune, tangerine.

Spices/Condiments/Sweeteners

Many spices have medicinal properties. Turmeric improves liver function. Ginger is anti-inflammatory and aids digestive health. Garlic improves immune health and is anti-inflammatory.

Many common food additives, such as guar gum and carrageenan, enhance the effects of lectins found in other foods and should be avoided.

SUPER BENEFICIAL	BENEFICIAL	NEUTRAL: Allowed Frequently	NEUTRAL: Allowed Infrequently	AVOID
Garlic	Horse-radish	Basil	Agar	Allspice
Ginger		Bay leaf	Apple pectin	Almond extract
Turmeric		Bergamot		

SUPER BENEFICIAL	BENEFICIAL	NEUTRAL: Allowed Frequently	NEUTRAL: Allowed Infrequently	AVOID
	Molasses (black-strap) Oregano Parsley	Caraway Cardamom Carob Chervil Chili powder Chive Cilantro (corian- der leaf) Cinnamon Clove Coriander Cream of tartar Cumin Dill Juniper Licorice root* Mace Marjoram Mint (all) Mustard (dry) Nutmeg Paprika Rosemary Saffron Sage Savory Sea salt Seaweeds	Arrowroot Chocolate Honey Maple syrup Mayon- naise Molasses Rice syrup Senna Soy sauce Sugar (brown/ white)	Anise Aspartame Barley malt Carrageenan Cornstarch Corn syrup Dextrose Fructose Gelatin (except veg- sourced) Guarana Gums (acacia/ Arabic/ guar) Invert sugar Ketchup Malto- dextrin MSG Pepper (black/ white) Pepper (cayenne) Pepper (pep- percorn/ red flakes) Pickle (all) Sucanat Tapioca Vinegar (all)

SUPER BENEFICIAL	BENEFICIAL	NEUTRAL: Allowed Frequently	NEUTRAL: Allowed Infrequently	AVOID
		Stevia		Worcester-shire sauce
		Tamari (wheat-free)		
		Tamarind		
		Tarragon		
		Thyme		
		Vanilla		
		Winter-green		
		Yeast (baker's/ brewer's)		

Special Variants: *Non-Secretor:* BENEFICIAL: bay leaf, yeast (brewer's); AVOID: agar, honey, juniper, maple syrup, rice syrup, sugar (brown/white).

*Do not use if you have high blood pressure.

Herbal Teas

Several herbal teas can be SUPER BENEFICIAL for Blood Type AB. Ginger contains pungent phenolic substances with pronounced antioxidative and anti-inflammatory activities. Echinacea is mildly stimulative to the immune system. Licorice root provides antiviral support and enhances cortisol modulation.

SUPER BENEFICIAL	BENEFICIAL	NEUTRAL: Allowed Frequently	NEUTRAL: Allowed Infrequently	AVOID
Echinacea	Alfalfa	Catnip	Senna	Aloe
Ginger	Burdock	Chickweed		Coltsfoot
Licorice root*	Chamomile	Dong quai		Corn silk
	Dandelion	Elder		Fenugreek

SUPER BENEFICIAL	BENEFICIAL	NEUTRAL: Allowed Frequently	NEUTRAL: Allowed Infrequently	AVOID
	Ginseng	Goldenseal		Gentian
	Hawthorn	Hore-hound		Hops
	Parsley	Mulberry		Linden
	Rosehip	Pepper-mint		Mullein
	Strawberry leaf	Raspberry leaf		Red clover
		Sage		Rhubarb
		Sarsa-parilla		Shepherd's purse
		Slippery elm		Skullcap
		Spearmint		
		St. John's wort		
		Thyme		
		Valerian		
		Vervain		
		White birch		
		White oak bark		
		Yarrow		
		Yellow dock		

Special Variants: None.

* Do not use if you have high blood pressure.

Miscellaneous Beverages

Green tea is a SUPER BENEFICIAL beverage for Blood Type AB because of its antioxidant and cardiovascular properties. Red wine contains gallic acid, trans-resveratrol, quercetin, and rutin—four phenolic compounds with potent antioxidant effects. Coffee should be avoided by Type AB, as it exacerbates allergies.

SUPER BENEFICIAL	BENEFICIAL	NEUTRAL: Allowed Frequently	NEUTRAL: Allowed Infrequently	AVOID
Tea (green)	Wine (red)	Seltzer Soda (club) Wine (white)	Beer	Coffee (reg/decaf) Liquor Soda (cola/diet/misc.) Tea, black (reg/decaf)
Special Variants: *Non-Secretor:* AVOID: beer.				

Supplements

THE BLOOD TYPE AB DIET offers abundant quantities of important nutrients, such as protein and iron. It is important to get as many nutrients as possible from fresh foods and use supplements only to fill in the minor deficiencies in your diet. The following supplement protocols are designed for Blood Type AB women to support health during and after menopause.

Note: If you are being treated for a medical condition, consult your doctor before taking any supplements.

Blood Type AB:
Basic Menopausal Support Protocol

Use this protocol for 6 weeks		
SUPPLEMENT	**ACTION**	**DOSAGE**
High-quality multiple vitamin complex (preferably blood type–specific)	Supports general health	As directed
Methylcobalamin (active vitamin B$_{12}$)	Supports nervous system	400 mcg, 1 capsule before bed
Black cohosh (*Cimicifuga racemosa)* standardized to 2.5% triterpene glycosides	Relieves menopausal symptoms, especially hot flashes	1–2 capsules, twice daily
Pyridoxine (vitamin B$_6$)	Supports nervous system health and mental function	50 mg daily
Sage tea (*Salvia officinalis*)	Relieves menopausal symptoms	1–2 cups daily

Blood Type AB:
Bone and Structural Support Protocol

Use this protocol for 6 weeks		
SUPPLEMENT	**ACTION**	**DOSAGE**
High-quality multiple vitamin complex (preferably blood type–specific)	Supports general health	As directed
Drynaria *spp*	In traditional Chinese medicine, one of the most important herbs that can be used to heal	50–250 mg, once or twice daily

SUPPLEMENT	ACTION	DOSAGE
	damaged bones and ligaments; literal Chinese name means "mender of shattered bones"; also appears to decrease the activity of bone-reabsorbing cells called osteoclasts.	
Vitamin A	Antioxidant immune support; necessary for bone health	10,000 IU, 1 capsule daily
Boron	Helps maintain healthy bones; enhances the metabolism of calcium, magnesium, copper, phosphorus, and vitamin D	1 mg, 1 capsule daily

Blood Type AB:
Cardiovascular Fitness Protocol

Use this protocol for 6 weeks		
SUPPLEMENT	ACTION	DOSAGE
Pantethine (active vitamin B$_5$)	Lowers cholesterol	500 mg, twice daily
Hawthorn	Improves coronary function; reduces angina	100 mg, twice daily
Standardized Chinese garlic extract (*Allium sativum*)	Lowers cholesterol	400 mg, twice daily
OPCs (oligomeric proanthocyanidins)	Have antioxidant effects	100 mg daily

Blood Type AB:
Skin Health and Vitality Protocol

Use this protocol for 4 weeks

SUPPLEMENT	ACTION	DOSAGE
OPCs (oligomeric proanthocyanidins)	Have antioxidant effects	100 mg daily
Vitamin A	Antioxidant immune support; necessary for bone health	10,000 IU, 1 capsule daily
Red clover (*Trifolium pratense*) tincture	Enhances collagen and serves as a natural blood cleanser; somewhat effective against hot flashes	5 drops, once or twice daily
(Non-secretors) Tea tree (*Leptospermum sp*) oil lotion (5%)	Treatment of acne, eczema, and fungal infections	Apply topically, twice daily, as needed

GENERAL RECOMMENDATIONS USABLE BY ALL GROUPS

Topical treatment with witch hazel (*Hamamelis virginiana*)
as needed

Topical treatment with marigold juice (*Calendula officinalis*)
as needed

Zinc, 15 mg: 1 capsule, twice daily

Niacinamide cream (4%): apply topically, twice daily

The Exercise Component

FOR BLOOD TYPE AB, overall fitness is achieved with a balance of moderate aerobic activity and mentally soothing, stress-reducing exercises. Below is a list of exercises that are recommended for Blood Type AB.

EXERCISE	DURATION	FREQUENCY
Martial arts	30–60 minutes	2–3 x week
Cycling	45–60 minutes	2–3 x week
Hiking	30–60 minutes	2–3 x week
Golf (no cart!)	60–90 minutes	2–3 x week
Walking	40–50 minutes	2–3 x week
Pilates	40–50 minutes	2–3 x week
Swimming	45 minutes	2–3 x week
Yoga	40–50 minutes	1–2 x week
T'ai Chi	40–50 minutes	1–2 x week

3 Steps to Effective Exercise

1. Warm up with stretching and flexibility moves before you start your aerobic exercise.
2. To achieve maximum cardiovascular benefits, work toward an elevated heart rate that is about 70 percent of your capacity. Once you reach the elevated rate, continue exercising to maintain that rate for twenty to thirty minutes. To calculate your maximum heart rate and performance level:
   - Subtract your age from 220.
   - Multiply the difference by .70 (or .60 if you are over age sixty). This is the high end of your performance.
   - Multiply the remainder by .50. This is the low end of your performance.
3. Finish each aerobic session with at least a five-minute cooldown of stretching and relaxation moves.

Getting Started: The First Month

IF YOU ARE NEW to the Blood Type Diet, the following guidelines will introduce you to the Blood Type AB regimen over a period of one month. Follow these recommendations as closely as possible, using a notebook to record your personal experiences with the diet. In addition to factors that are measurable in laboratory tests, take the time to note changes in your energy levels, sleep patterns, digestion, and over-all well-being.

I advise that you keep a daily journal of your symptoms, the times they occur, and the circumstances. This will help you better manage them. If you are experiencing perimenopause, keep a record of your cycles and the changes you notice.

Blood Type AB Diet Checklist
for the Menopausal Woman

Derive your protein primarily from sources other than red meat. ☐

Eliminate chicken from your diet. ☐

Eat soy foods and seafood as your primary protein. ☐

Include modest amounts of cultured dairy foods in your diet, but limit fresh milk products. ☐

Don't overdo the grains, especially wheat-derived foods. Avoid corn flour altogether. ☐

Eat lots of BENEFICIAL fruits and vegetables, especially those high in antioxidants and fiber. ☐

Avoid coffee, but drink two to three cups of green tea every day. ☐

Week 1

Blood Type Diet and Supplements

- Eliminate your most harmful AVOID foods—chicken, corn, buckwheat, most shellfish, and lectin-activated beans.
- Include your most important BENEFICIAL foods frequently throughout the week. For example, have soy-based foods 5 times, and omega-3-rich fish 3 to 4 times, with lots of BENEFICIAL vegetables and fruit.

- Incorporate at least 1 SUPER BENEFICIAL into your daily diet. For example, eat slices of fresh pineapple over yogurt, or sprinkle walnuts on a salad.
- If you're a coffee drinker, begin to wean yourself by cutting your daily consumption in half. Substitute green tea.

Exercise Regimen

- Plan to exercise at least 4 days this week, for 45 minutes each day.

  2 days: walking or light aerobic activity

  2 days: yoga or T'ai Chi

- Use your journal to detail the time, activity, and distance. Note the number of repetitions for each exercise.

■ WEEK 1 SUCCESS STRATEGY ■
Get the Most Accurate Mammogram

There is a lot of concern about whether women are getting the most accurate mammogram readings. Here are some steps you can take to improve the accuracy of your breast cancer screening test:

- Try to go to the same breast cancer screening clinic year after year.
- If you change your clinic, try to obtain the X-ray film so there will be a point of comparison.
- If you are still menstruating, wait until after your period to get a mammogram. Your breast tissue undergoes changes during your period.
- Alert the radiologist if you take hormone replacement therapy, which can make your breast tissue denser and harder to read. Some radiologists use ultrasound in combination with mammograms to get the most accurate reading.

Week 2

Blood Type Diet and Supplements

- Begin to eliminate the next level of AVOID foods—grains, vegetables, and fruits that react poorly with Type AB blood.
- Eat 2 to 3 BENEFICIAL proteins every day.

- Continue to incorporate SUPER BENEFICIAL foods into your daily diet.
- Choose the NEUTRAL foods listed as "Allowed Frequently" over those listed "Allowed Infrequently."
- If you're a coffee drinker, continue to cut your coffee intake, replacing it with green tea.
- Manage your mealtimes to aid proper digestion. Avoid eating on the run. Make your meals relaxing, sit-down affairs. Eat slowly and chew thoroughly to encourage digestive secretions.

Exercise Regimen

- Continue to exercise at least 4 days this week, for 45 minutes each day.

  2 days: walking or light aerobic activity

  2 days: yoga or T'ai Chi
- If your work is sedentary, get in the habit of taking a couple of "movement" breaks during the day. Walk around the block or up and down stairs.

▪ WEEK 2 SUCCESS STRATEGY ▪
Dry Skin Brushing

Dry skin brushing is a method of daily hygiene that has many benefits and has been around for a long time. The skin is a major organ of the body that functions as protection and as a means of elimination. What daily skin brushing will do:

- Removes dried, dead cells that block the pores of the skin, allowing the skin to breathe easier and increasing its ability to protect and eliminate the waste products of metabolism.
- Increases circulation of the blood and lymph vessels that lie close to the surface just under the skin. The blood, fluid, and its contents are returned to the heart for redistribution and/or elimination.
- Increases the nutrients to the skin. By clearing out stagnant materials, there is an increased oxygen/carbon dioxide exchange, and other nutrients, vitamins, minerals, enzymes, etc., are also brought to the area.
- Removes waste products of cellular metabolism through the blood vessels and sweating.

- Decreases the workload on the rest of the body in regard to circulation and elimination.
- Warms the skin.

PROCEDURE

Skin brushing should be done with a natural- or nylon-bristle body brush before the bath or the shower but can replace the bath if no water is available. It is suggested the brushing be done toward the heart; start with the lower limbs, arms, back, then the front of the body, using a moderate pressure with short strokes upward and inward. If you have a soft-complexion brush, the face can be done as well, using more circular motions. Strokes should bring a slight pink color or tingling sensation to the skin—never bruising, scraping, bleeding, or pain. One time through for each body area is sufficient.

AVOID SKIN BRUSHING IF

- You have delicate skin.
- You have easily damaged skin.
- You have an open wound.
- You have known malignancies of the skin or lymph system.

Week 3

Blood Type Diet and Supplements

- When you plan your meals for week 3, choose BENEFICIAL foods to replace NEUTRAL foods whenever possible.
- Eliminate all remaining AVOID foods.
- Liberally incorporate SUPER BENEFICIAL foods into your daily diet.
- Completely wean yourself from coffee, substituting green tea.

Exercise Regimen

- Continue to exercise at least 4 days this week, for 45 minutes each day.

  2 days: walking or light aerobic activity

  2 days: yoga or T'ai Chi

■ WEEK 3 SUCCESS STRATEGY ■
Cool Down the Hot Flashes

Here are some natural ways to keep your hot flashes in check:

- Wear layered clothing so you can remove items if you feel overheated during the day.
- Avoid caffeine and alcohol; they can trigger flashes in some women.
- Minimize your use of hot spices like cayenne pepper.
- Certain medications, such as those prescribed to lower blood pressure, can bring on flashes. If this is a problem, ask your doctor to prescribe a different formula.
- A tepid shower can help bring down body temperature.

Week 4

Blood Type Diet

- Continue at the week 3 level, focusing on BENEFICIAL and SUPER BENEFICIAL foods.

Exercise Regimen

- Continue at the week 3 level.
- Review your progress, noting in your journal improvements in strength and flexibility. Determine which exercise regimen has worked for you, including time of day, setting, and activity level.

■ WEEK 4 SUCCESS STRATEGY ■
Maximize Energy with the Right Eating Schedule

For Blood Type AB, the timing of your meals can be almost as important as what you eat. This is particularly true if you're trying to lose weight. The following are helpful guidelines:

- Never skip meals. You won't be "saving" calories, as the metabolic reaction will foil your efforts.

- Make breakfast your most important protein-rich meal of the day. The result will be an efficient metabolism all day long.
- Eat on a sliding scale: big breakfast, medium lunch, small dinner.
- Resist the late-night munchies, but if you have problems regulating blood sugar, have a small protein snack—yogurt or soy milk—before bedtime.

Appendices

A Simple
Definition
of Terms

agglutination: Clumping, or "gluing" together. Agglutination is one means by which the immune system defends against foreign matter and toxins, notably against lectins and opposing blood type material.

andropause: The term used to describe "male menopause"—the hormonal, physiological, and chemical changes that occur with age.

antibody: The product of the immune system when it is stimulated by specific antigens. There are many classes of antibodies, among them "agglutinins," which isolate foreign substances by clumping them together so that they may be eliminated. Blood Types O, A, and B manufacture antibodies to other blood types. Blood Type AB, the universal recipient, manufactures no antibodies to other blood types.

antigen: A chemical that provokes an immune system antibody response. The blood type "ID" present on the blood cells, identified as type A or B, is one example. A type AB cell has both of these antigens. The blood type having no antigen is described as O—or "Zero." As we age, it is to our advantage to shore up our store of circulating anti–blood type antigens, as lower levels mean increased susceptibility to diseases arising from substances and organisms bearing opposing antigens.

antioxidant: Antioxidants are important, naturally occurring nutrients that help maintain health by slowing the destructive aging process of cellular molecules such as free radicals. As cells function normally in the body, they produce damaged molecules—called free radicals. Antioxidants help prevent widespread cellular destruction by willingly donating components to stabilize free radicals, and are thus known to moderate the oxidation, or aging, process in human cells, by lowering free radical levels. Many healthy foods are rich sources of antioxidants, including the element selenium and the vitamins C, E, and A. Vitamins C and E and many plants and plant-derived substances such as green tea, quercetin, larch arabinogalactan, and milk thistle are potent antioxidants.

autoimmune diseases: Diseases generated when the cells that normally defend the body against infections mistakenly attack its own cells, tissues, and organs.

blood type: The term commonly used to refer to the ABO blood group system. Originally used primarily to determine suitable blood and organ donor–recipient matches, ABO type determines many of the digestive and immunological characteristics of the body, as well as susceptibility to the diseases arising from infection, immune suppression, and digestive impairment. It is also one of the tools used by anthropologists to establish the origins, socioeconomic development, and movements of ancient peoples.

catecholamines: Adrenaline and noradrenaline, hormones released from the adrenal glands in response to stress.

cortisol: A catabolic hormone produced by the adrenal glands in response to trauma. Cortisol breaks down muscle tissue and converts the proteins from the tissue into energy.

DHEA (dehydroepiandrosterone): A steroid hormone made from cholesterol by the adrenal glands. DHEA enhances the activity of other hormones and contributes to energy levels, libido, and metabolic balance. It sharply declines after menopause.

estradiol: See estrogen.

estriol: See estrogen.

estrogen: The primary female sex hormone, estrogen occurs in estrogenic compounds: estradiol, estrone, and estriol. *Estradiol* is the most potent estrogen. In women it is responsible for growth of the breast and reproductive epithelia, maturation of long bones, and development of the secondary sex characteristics. Estradiol is produced mainly by the ovaries with secondary production by the adrenal glands and conversion of steroid precursors into estrogens in fat tissue. *Estrone* is produced primarily from androstenedione originating from the gonads or the adrenal cortex. After menopause, estrone levels increase, possibly due to increased conversion of androstenedione to estrone. *Estriol* is the weakest of the three estrogens, produced almost exclusively during pregnancy, and is the major estrogen produced in the normal human fetus. Estriol is thought to be less carcinogenic than estradiol and estrone and can be used at low doses and in topical preparations for the relief of menopausal symptoms.

estrone: See estrogen.

glutathione: A small molecule made inside almost every cell, from its three constituent amino acids: glycine, glutamate, and cysteine. Glutathione is the major antioxidant produced by the cell, protecting it from free radicals.

hyperthyroidism: The overactive thyroid, conventionally treated with long-term antithyroid drugs or thyroidectomy, partial removal or destruction with radioactive iodine or surgery. Thyroid diseases show a preference for Blood Type O individuals. While medical intervention is recommended in the case of hyperthyroid function, reducing the types and amount of anti–blood type lectins present in the diet, especially those found in certain grains and legumes, can be of great help in resolving these conditions.

hypothyroidism: Underproduction of thyroid hormone, thyroxine (t3) and/or free triiodothyronine (t4). Conventionally treated by hormone replacement therapy. Thyroid conditions often respond favorably to a blood type–appropriate diet.

immune system: The physiological determination of and response to "self" and "non-self" accomplished through the action of many organs and cells throughout the body, essential to the preservation of its health and integrity.

lectins: Proteins that attach to preferred receptors in the human body. Food lectins are often blood type-specific. A lectin's action may initiate agglutination, inflammation, the abnormal proliferation of cells of the immune and nervous systems, or insulin resistance, depending upon the type of cells targeted. Abundant in the vegetable kingdom, lectins are fewer in number and type among animal foods.

menopause: A stage in life when a woman stops having her monthly period. By definition, a woman is menopausal after her periods have stopped for one year. Menopause typically occurs in a woman's late forties to early fifties. It is a normal part of aging, marking the end of a woman's reproductive years. Women who have their ovaries surgically removed undergo "sudden" menopause.

metabolism: The aggregate of physical and chemical processes by which organisms maintain life, in the opposing functions of building tissue (anabolism) and breaking down tissue and foreign matter to be used as fuel (catabolism).

nitric oxide: A short-lived molecule crucial to the regulation of the central nervous system.

perimenopause: The term used to describe the time of transition between a woman's reproductive years and when menstruation ceases completely.

polyamines: A group of cell components (putrescine, spermidine, and spermine) that are important in the regulation of cell proliferation and cell differentiation. There is also evidence suggesting a role for polyamines in programmed cell death. Although their exact functions have not yet been identified, it is clear that polyamines play important roles in a number of cellular processes.

progesterone: A female hormone secreted by the corpus luteum after ovulation, which prepares the lining of the uterus for a fertilized egg. At menopause, progesterone levels decline to nearly zero.

testosterone: The primary male sex hormone, also produced in lesser amounts in women's ovaries and adrenal glands. Testosterone builds muscle and bone and is responsible for libido.

FAQs: Blood Type and Menopause

I am Blood Type A, and I have been following your dietary guidelines with wonderful results. I've recently stopped using hormone replacement therapy, and I wonder if you could make recommendations for Type A menopausal women. In addition to following the dietary program, what should we do to relieve symptoms such as hot flashes and to protect ourselves from bone loss and cardiovascular problems?

Herbal remedies such as black cohosh, dong quai, and primrose oil are generally fine for menopausal Type A women. The supplement protocols in the Type A chapter contain additional information.

I am a 55-year-old Type O non-secretor and have been on the Blood Type Diet for two years with great success. Osteoporosis runs in my family; both my mother and grandmother have severely curved spines. How can I avoid that fate?

The Type O Diet and exercise plan is your best road to bone

health. Here are some other things that will help. Limit salt and caffeine, as they have been linked to bone loss. Soft drinks, which have high levels of phosphoric acid, may be harmful to bones. Smoking leads to increased bone loss. For this and many other health reasons, it should be avoided.

Calcium supplements help prevent and treat weak bones. Many adults take 800 to 1,200 mg of calcium per day. Vitamin D increases calcium absorption. Since calcium may reduce absorption of magnesium and zinc, which are important nutrients for preventing osteoporosis, it may be prudent to also supplement these minerals: 25 mg of zinc and 200 to 400 mg of magnesium per day are reasonable amounts. Copper helps in bone synthesis: A recent study found that 3 mg of copper added per day may help prevent bone loss.

At our Web site (www.dadamo.com) you can learn about a new mineral formula that contains a special form of calcium derived from the small red seaweed called maerl, found only in the isolated areas off the pristine coast of northwest Ireland. Of all sources of calcium, maerl has one of the lowest levels of undesirable contaminants. Its superior buffering capacity allows maerl-based calcium to maintain very high rates of absorption.

I am sixty-two years old, and I feel as if I've lost the battle of my spreading waistline. Is it really possible to avoid abdominal fat at my age?

Yes! In a recent study published in the *Journal of the American Medical Association*, postmenopausal women who began an exercise program of brisk walking or cycling lowered levels of abdominal fat by about 6 percent and lost weight, regardless of body weight or age. In the study, Dr. Anne McTiernan and her colleagues, from the Fred Hutchinson Cancer Research Center in Seattle, Washington, assessed the outcomes of 168 sedentary women, between fifty and seventy years of age, who were randomized to perform moderate-intensity exercises or stretching. All of the women had a body mass index over 25. The exercisers walked on a treadmill or cycled on a stationary bicycle for at least forty-five minutes, five days a week, for one year. Weight training was recommended but not required. Women in the control group performed a series of stretching exercises one day a week for the year.

The most active women, or those who exercised more than three hours and fifteen minutes a week, lost about 7 percent of intra-abdominal fat, compared with a loss of 6 percent among intermediate exercisers, as measured by a CT scan. The study found that those who exercised less than two hours and fifteen minutes a week lost 3.4 percent of their intra-abdominal fat, while women in the control group gained 0.1 percent intra-abdominal fat. Body weight decreased by an average of 1.3 kg in the exercise group, while body weight rose slightly in the control group.

I read that taking vitamin A supplements might cause bone loss. Is this true?

There were early studies that seemed to draw this conclusion, but they have been deemed inaccurate based on newer studies. It may well be that vitamin A suffered from a form of guilt by association, as the main sources of vitamin A in the diet are vitamin A–fortified foods such as margarine, sugary breakfast cereals, and milk—all of which can contribute to osteoporosis for reasons entirely unrelated to vitamin A.

Why are different exercises recommended for people with different blood types?

The exercise recommendations are focused on improving total systemic health, mainly the functioning of the organs, glands, and immune and circulatory systems of the body, as opposed to building muscle tissue (which can be viewed as a pleasant side effect). What strenuous exercise does for Type O, yoga does for Type A, and aerobic exercise does for Types B and AB. Exercise recommendations are made with a general bias toward a person with a sedentary lifestyle. The link between blood type, stress, and exercise is discussed in *Live Right 4 Your Type: The Individualized Prescription for Maximizing Health, Metabolism, and Vitality in Every Stage of Your Life*. See appendix C for details.

I am a forty-eight-year-old female with Type AB blood. I have a strong family history of uterine fibroids for several generations. Many relatives had hysterectomies. I do not want to go this course. My periods are heavy and painful. I see very little written about this common premenopausal problem in women. Any advice? I am a month into the diet.

Uterine fibroids are benign tumors of the uterus. They are typically nonsymptomatic unless embedded in the lining, when they can cause heavy bleeding at menses. They are more common for Types A and AB, probably due to the fact that cellular growth factors responsible for the proliferation of uterine tissue can be stimulated by the A antigen. It has also been shown that hyperlastic (rapidly growing) endometrial tissue is heavily infiltrated with blood type antigens, whereas normal endometrial tissue is not.

I would suggest lowering the effects of growth-stimulating polyamines, which can accelerate cellular turnover. You can achieve this by eating plenty of soy foods and by avoiding highly processed or frozen foods. You can also try two herbal remedies traditionally used for treating uterine fibroids—capsella, or shepherd's purse, and chlorophyll (the green pigment in plants). As with any medical condition characterized by excess bleeding, it is prudent to make sure that the cause of the bleeding is not from more serious reasons. Be sure you consult your doctor.

I am a fifty-five-year-old Blood Type O woman with a long history of recurrent major depression. My naturopath has recommended St. John's wort. Why do you discourage this supplement for Blood Type O?

Blood Type O has lower levels of the enzyme MAO, and St. John's wort is an MAO inhibitor. This may explain why many Type Os on St. John's wort say they feel "weird" or have disturbing dreams. I have found, however, that Blood Type Os with mild to moderate depression benefit from the amino acid tyrosine, which can boost dopamine levels, or the Russian adaptogenic herb rhodiola, which helps modulate adrenaline and dopamine levels in the brain. Strangely enough, studies have shown that in men with a recent history of heart attack, those who were Type O blood tested much higher on the scale of "Type A behavior" than the other blood types, which would make eliminating excess adrenaline even more important.

Should I avoid genetically engineered food?

Yes! Genetic engineering moves lectin molecules from one species to another. Since lectins are the molecules that interact with our blood types, an okay food can easily become an AVOID. Currently, the only way to safely avoid "GE" foods is to choose organic.

Resources
and Products

General

American College of Obstetricians and Gynecologists (ACOG)
409 12th Street, SW
Box 96920
Washington, DC 20090-6920
202-638-5577
http:www.acog.org

North American Menopause Society
P.O. Box 94527
Cleveland, OH 44101
440-442-7550
1-800-774-5342
http:www.menopause.org

National Institute on Aging Information Center
P.O. Box 8057
Gaithersburg, MD 20898-8057
1-800-222-2225
1-800-222-4225 (TTY)
E-mail: niainfo@jbs1.com
http:www.nia.nih.gov

The National Institute on Aging offers free information on menopause and osteoporosis.

Additional information about menopausal hormones and the Women's Health Initiative is available on the National Institutes of Health (NIH) Web site—www.nih. Additional information about the WHI study is available on the Women's Health Initiative Participant Web site at http://www.whi.org.

The Institute for Human Individuality
Southwest College of Naturopathic Medicine
2140 E. Broadway Road
Tempe, AZ 85282
480-858-9100
www.ifhi-online.org

The Institute for Human Individuality is under the 501c3 status of Southwest College of Naturopathic Medicine. Its prime goal is to foster research in the expanding area of human nutrigenomics. Nutrigenomics seeks to provide a molecular understanding for how common dietary chemicals affect health by altering the expression or structure of an individual's genetic makeup. (IFHI is currently conducting a twelve-week randomized, double-blind, controlled trial implementing the Blood Type Diet to determine its effects on the outcomes of patients with rheumatoid arthritis.)

Blood Type–Specific Resources

Dr. Peter D'Adamo

The D'Adamo Naturopathic Clinic in Wilton, Connecticut, blends time-honored natural healing techniques with state-of-the-art diagnostics. The clinic staff is comprised of naturopathic physicians (ND) working with medical doctors (MD), nurses (RN), and other licensed health professionals, all under the precepts and guidance of Dr. Peter D'Adamo. To find out more or to schedule an appointment, please contact:

The D'Adamo Naturopathic Center
213 Danbury Road
Wilton, CT 06897
203-834-7500

www.dadamo.com

The World Wide Web has proven to be a valuable venue for exploring and applying the tenets of the Blood Type Diet and lifestyle. Since January 1997, hundreds of thousands have visited the site to participate in the ABO chat groups, to peruse the scientific archives, to share experiences and recipes, and to learn more about the science of blood type.

Blood Type Specialty Products and Supplements

North American Pharmacal, Inc., is the official distributor of Blood Type specialty products. The product line includes supplements, books, tapes, teas, meal replacement bars, cosmetics, and support material that make eating and living right for your type easier. Stop by our Web store at www.4yourtype.com or order toll-free at 877-ABO TYPE.

Home Blood-Typing Kits

North American Pharmacal, Inc., is the official distributor of Home
Blood Type Testing Kits. Each kit costs $9.95 (plus shipping and han-
dling) and is a single-use, disposable, educational device capable of de-
termining one individual's ABO and Rhesus (Rh) blood type. Results
are obtained within about four to five minutes. If you have several
friends or family members who need to learn their blood type, you will
need to order a separate home blood-typing kit for each individual.

The Blood Type Library

The following books are available in bookstores, health-food stores, se-
lected grocery and specialty stores, on the Web, and through North
American Pharmacal.

Eat Right 4 Your Type
*The Individualized Diet Solution to Staying Healthy, Living Longer, and
Achieving Your Ideal Weight*
By Dr. Peter J. D'Adamo, with Catherine Whitney
G. P. Putnam's Sons, 1996
   The original Blood Type Diet book, with over two million copies
sold in more than sixty-five languages.

Cook Right 4 Your Type
The Practical Kitchen Companion to Eat Right 4 Your Type
By Dr. Peter J. D'Adamo, with Catherine Whitney
G. P. Putnam's Sons, 1998 (Berkley Trade Paperback, 1999)
   Includes over two hundred original recipes, thirty-day meal plans,
and guidelines for each blood type.

Live Right 4 Your Type
*The Individualized Prescription for Maximizing Health, Metabolism, and Vi-
tality in Every Stage of Your Life*
By Dr. Peter J. D'Adamo, with Catherine Whitney
G. P. Putnam's Sons, 2001
   A total health and lifestyle plan based on the individual variations
observed for each blood type. Includes new research on the mind-body
connection and the importance of blood type secretor status.

Eat Right 4 Your Type Complete Blood Type Encyclopedia
By Dr. Peter J. D'Adamo, with Catherine Whitney
Riverhead Books, 2002

The A-to-Z reference guide for the blood type connection to symptoms, diseases, conditions, medications, vitamins, supplements, herbs, and food.

4 Your Type Pocket Guides
Blood Type, Food, Beverage and Supplement Lists
By Peter J. D'Adamo, with Catherine Whitney
Berkley Books, 2002

The Eat Right 4 Your Type Portable and Personal Blood Type Guides are pocket-sized and user-friendly. They serve as a handy reference tool while shopping, cooking, and eating out. Each book contains the food, beverage, and supplement list for each blood type plus handy tips and ideas for incorporating the Blood Type Diet into your daily life.

Eat Right 4 Your Baby
The Individualized Guide to Fertility and Maximum Health During Pregnancy, Nursing, and Your Baby's First Year
By Dr. Peter J. D'Adamo, with Catherine Whitney
G. P. Putnam's Sons, 2003

An invaluable guide for couples looking to combine the best of naturopathic and blood type science to maximize the health of mother and baby—with practical blood type–specific guidelines for achieving a healthy state before pregnancy, eating and living right during pregnancy, and continuing in good health during baby's first year.

Dr. Peter J. D'Adamo's Eat Right 4 (for) Your Type Health Library
Aging: Fight It with the Blood Type Diet ®
Allerigies: Fight Them with the Blood Type Diet ®
Arthritis: Fight It with the Blood Type Diet ®
Cancer: Fight It with the Blood Type Diet ®
Cardiovascular Disease: Fight It with the Blood Type Diet ®
Diabetes: Fight It with the Blood Type Diet ®
Fatigue: Fight It with the Blood Type Diet ®

Index

OPCs (oligomeric proanthocyandins), 125–26, 157–58
Oranges, 51
Osteoporosis, 11, 99, 175–77

Pantethine (active Vit B_5), 92, 157
Pantothenic acid (Vit. B_5), 60, 126
Peanut oil, 44, 76
Perimenopause, 8, 173
Peroxidase, 122
Phenolic acids, 122
Phenylalanine, 81
Phosphorus, 105, 107, 139
Phytochemicals, 51, 77, 143
Phytoestrogens, 27–28, 75, 79, 143, 147
Pineapple, 150
Plums, 51, 83, 117
Polyamines, 139, 173, 178
Polyphenols, 43, 57, 109, 123, 142
Poultry. See Meat/poultry
Premarin, 12–13, 26
Prempro, 13
Probiotics, 31, 60, 66, 92
Products, 183–86
Progesterone, 8, 14, 173
Progesterone creams, 28
Provera, 12–13
Prunes, 83
Pyridoxine (vitamin B_6), 90, 156

Quercetin, 89, 155

Red clover, 158
Red snapper, 39
Red wine, 57, 89, 123, 155
Resources, 181–83
Rhodiola, 178
Risk factors, 10–12
RNA (ribonucleic acid), 30
Rosehip tea, 87
Rosmarinic acid, 121
Rutin, 89, 155

Safflower oil, 44, 142
Sage, 121–22
Sage tea, 156
St. John's wort, 178–79

Salmon, 71, 105, 139
Sardines, 71, 105, 139
Sarsaparilla, 126
Sarsaparilla tea, 56
Seafood. See Fish/seafood
Seaweed, 49, 176
Secretors, 19–20, 107, 136
Seeds. See Nuts/seeds
Sesame oil, 109, 142
Sex drive, 10
Shiitake mushrooms, 114, 147
Skin changes, 10
Skin health/vitality protocol
    Blood Type A, 92–93
    Blood Type AB, 158
    Blood Type B, 126
    Blood Type O, 60
Sleep problems, 10, 98–99
Soda, 57
SOD (superoxide dismutase), 122
Sorghum, 47
Soy beans, 27, 46, 78, 111
Soy isoflavones, 27, 46, 78, 90, 144–45
Spices/condiments/sweeteners
    Blood Type A, 85–87
    Blood Type AB, 151–53
    Blood Type B, 119–21
    Blood Type O, 53–55
Spinach, 49, 81, 114, 147
Sprouted grain breads, 47, 113, 146
Squalenes, 43, 109, 142
Squaw vine, 90
Standardized Chinese garlic extract, 157
Starches. See Grains/starches
Stress, 29–30, 97
Stress-reducing exercise, 127, 158
Sunflower oil, 109
Super foods
    Blood Type A, 68–69
    Blood Type AB, 136
    Blood Type B, 102
    Blood Type O, 36
Supersoy, 27, 78
Supplements, 30–31, 175
    Blood Type A, 89–93
    Blood Type AB, 155–58